Pain As Human Experience

COMPARATIVE STUDIES OF
HEALTH SYSTEMS AND MEDICAL CARE

For a complete list of titles in this series, please contact the
Sales Department
University of California Press
2120 Berkeley Way
Berkeley, CA 94720

Pain as Human Experience: An Anthropological Perspective

EDITED BY

Mary-Jo DelVecchio Good,
Paul E. Brodwin, Byron J. Good,
Arthur Kleinman

UNIVERSITY OF CALIFORNA PRESS
Berkeley   Los Angeles   London

This book is a print-on-demand volume. It is manufactured using toner in place of ink. Type and images may be less sharp than the same material seen in traditionally printed University of California Press editions.

University of California Press
Berkeley and Los Angeles, California
University of California Press, Ltd.
London, England
Copyright © 1992 by The Regents of the University of California

First Paperback Printing 1994

Library of Congress Cataloging-in-Publication Data
Pain as human experience: an anthropological perspective / edited by
    Mary-Jo D. Good . . . [et al.].
        p.   cm.—(Comparative studies of health systems and medical
    care; no. 31)
    Includes bibliographical references and index.
    ISBN 0-520-07512-9
    1. Medical anthropology.   2. Pain—Social aspects.   I. Good,
    Mary-Jo D. (Mary-Jo DelVecchio)   II. Series.
    GN296.P35   1992
    306.4'61—dc20   91-14044
                                                                 CIP

Printed in the United States of America

CONTENTS

ACKNOWLEDGMENTS

The authors express their gratitude to the National Science Foundation for a research grant (No. 83-09816) to study chronic pain from an anthropological perspective, and to the National Institute of Mental Health for funds for a research training program in clinically relevant medical anthropology (MH 18006), several of whose members contributed to research covered in this volume. The research on pain in China, described in chapter 7, was funded by grants to Arthur Kleinman from the Social Science Research Council and the Committee on Scholarly Communication with the People's Republic of China of the National Academy of Sciences.

For assistance in preparing the manuscript, we thank Joan Gillespie, Barbara Graham, and Margaret Zaldivar.

We are particularly grateful to the many individuals suffering from chronic pain who participated in this research and who generously contributed their time and thoughts through the interview process. We hope that what we have learned through their narratives will contribute to the development of a patient-centered orientation to problems created by the experience of chronic pain and will improve the quality of health care for pain patients. We also appreciate the assistance of the clinicians who contributed to the studies discussed in this book. For reasons of confidentiality, we cannot thank them by name or acknowledge their institutions.

CHAPTER ONE

Pain as Human Experience: An Introduction

Arthur Kleinman, Paul E. Brodwin, Byron J. Good,
Mary-Jo DelVecchio Good

Pain is a ubiquitous feature of human experience. Acute pain, lasting minutes or hours, is reported at some time by virtually all adults in North American society, across the span of ethnic groups and social classes, of age and gender. It is the single most frequent complaint brought to the offices of physicians in North America (Osterweis et al. 1987). Pain is also a focus of serious attention in the literate medical traditions of China, India, and Islamic cultures (Brihaye et al. 1987). Ethnographers, physicians, and public health experts describe pain complaints for a great variety of societies. Neuroscientists regard pain as a salient feature of the nervous system.[1] It is thus reasonable to assume that pain is a universal feature of the human condition.

At the same time, the cultural elaboration of pain involves categories, idioms, and modes of experience that are greatly diverse. Ohnuki-Tierney, for example, describes complaints among Sakhalin Ainu of Japan as including "bear headaches" that "sound" like the heavy steps of a bear; "deer headaches" that feel like the much lighter sounds of running deer; and "woodpecker headaches" that feel like a woodpecker pounding into the trunk of a tree (Ohnuki-Tierney 1981:49). Ots (1990) describes a common experience of headache among Chinese as characterized by a painful dizziness or vertigo—a complaint that is an embodiment of the traditional Chinese medical category of imbalance as the proximate cause of ill health. Abad and Boyce (1979:34) report that Latinos in North America distinguish *dolor de cabeza* (headache) and *dolor del cerebro* (brainache) as two distinctive experiences and disorders. Headache is a common complaint of Latino patients who suffer *nervios*, a core idiom and syndrome of distress in Latin American cultures (Guarnaccia and Farias 1988). Ebigbo (1982) indicates that Nigerians complain of a wide range of specific pains, using language that would be considered potential indicators of psychosis in this country: "it seems as if pepper were put into my head," "things like ants keep on creeping in various parts of my brain," or "by merely touching parts of my brain it hurts."

Medical anthropologists frequently cite Zborowski's (1952, 1969) studies of the role of ethnicity in the stylization of pain expression—studies conducted in a veterans' hospital in New York state—as the *locus classicus* of serious scholarly anthropological interest in the relationship of pain and culture. While this claim may not be historically accurate—W. H. R. Rivers, Erwin Ackerknecht, and others preceded Zborowski with inquiries into this topic—it is appropriate with respect to magnitude of influence. Zborowski drew upon differences in worldview, including orientation to time, to explain the reactions of "old Yankees," Irish, Jews, and Italians to bodily pain. Nowadays, his writing seems like a quaint anachronism. The cultural stereotypes, elaborated from a study of male veterans, are elevated above particularities of person, gender, and situation. They are ahistorical and unchanging. The peculiar qualities of the sting and throb of pain affecting a particular person—with a unique story, living in a certain community and historical period, and above all with fears, longings, aspirations—are washed away in the ethnic stereotype: Yankees are continent; Jews and Italians are expressive; Jews are more concerned with the future significance of their pain; Italians, focused on the present, are simply relieved that the pain has gone away.

We blush to read these descriptions today. They create cardboard characters instead of describing real people. For all their good intentions and the residuum of group differences they may (or may not) capture, these ethnic caricatures hold little interpretive value; they are even dehumanizing (see Migliore 1989; Lipton and Marbach 1984; Craig and Wyckoff 1987). Zborowski's important accomplishment was to open the study of pain to cultural comparisons and to illustrate ways by which meanings shape behavior; however, his work led a generation of social scientists and health professionals into a conceptual and methodological cul-de-sac. The problem is more than an inadequate conception of ethnicity and the acceptance of a superficial level of understanding. His approach to cultural analysis fails to address pain as an intimate feature of lived experience of individuals in the context of their local social world and historical epoch.

Fabrega and Tyma (1976a, 1976b), by contrast, recreate the relationship of pain and culture as a greatly complex knot of bodily, psychological, and philosophical conundrums. Using evidence from neurobiology, hermeneutics, psychosomatic medicine, and ultimately epistemology, they portray the ramifying connections between peripheral pain fibers transmitting messages from sensory receptors to the central nervous system, where they are modulated by hormonal, affective, and perceptual processes—all influenced by cultural categories and social relations. Fabrega and Tyma thereby create a

subject matter so densely interrelated and multileveled and of such astonishing complexity that the reader (social scientist or health scientist) must
despair at ever grasping the processes that mediate a pounding headache or
that transform a social stigma into the nauseating cramping of abdominal
distress. With such a vast network of "variables," whose resonances and
results are so poorly charted, it is not surprising that researchers have defined (or created) a subject matter they can actually study with available
conceptual and methodological approaches. Thus arises the recent interest in
chronic pain and the diverse disciplinary approaches to its study.

CHRONIC PAIN

Unlike acute pain, chronic pain (lasting months or years) is not a ubiquitous
experience. Nor has it been shown to be universal, crossing cultures and historical epochs. But it is not infrequent either. In the United States, chronic
pain is among the most frequent reasons for disablement (Osterweis et al.
1987). A substantial portion of disability payments goes to those with chronic
pain complaints. While only approximately 7 percent of individuals who experience low back pain in the workplace go on to develop chronic symptoms
that impair family functioning and work performance, those individuals who
do develop chronic pain syndromes occupy much of the time and receive
a disproportionately large percentage of the funds of disability programs
(ibid.).

Chronic pain syndromes highlight the fault lines of society. Patients with
chronic pain on the Social Security Administration's (SSA) Disability Insurance Program are more likely to be relatively unskilled workers with limited
education from poor, inner-city ethnic groups than middle-class professionals. While the former probably experience greater biomechanical stress in
their workaday world, social factors also significantly affect both their pain
and disability. Increasing unemployment, for example, is directly correlated
with increasing disability claims and numbers of claimants who enter the
disability rolls (Berkowitz 1987). As a result, chronic pain has become associated with income redistribution (Stone 1984). Social forces influence not only
who develops chronic pain and who is disabled by it but also who responds to
treatment and rehabilitation and who becomes permanently disabled. Local
conditions in the workplace, for example, turn out to be better predictors of
who among the disabled will return to work than biomedical indexes (Yelin
et al. 1980). Heretofore, the largest share of social science research on chronic
pain has focused on working-class samples for whom work disability was the
central issue. With expenditures of public funds going to more than forty-two
million noninstitutionalized adults in the United States in 1977 as a source of
family income, more than twelve million of whom were disabled, and with
one out of four of the severely disabled suffering from a job-related condition,

it is not all that surprising that this has been the emphasis (Work Disability in the United States 1980).

What is surprising is the uncertain status of chronic pain in biomedicine and in the biomedically oriented disability system in the United States. The concept is so poorly defined that chronic pain syndromes lack official status within the standard biomedical taxonomy. The American Psychiatric Association's *DSM-III* category of "Psychogenic Pain"—subsequently dropped in *DSM-III-R*—was unacceptable because physicians and psychologists find relatively few cases of pain in which the etiology is clearly and solely psychological. What one does find is a profusion of discrete conditions—low back pain, chest pain (without heart or lung pathology), functional bowel syndrome, headaches, and so on—without agreement on a unifying rubric. Although chronic pain is one of the most frequent conditions brought to the SSA's Disability Insurance Program, that program does not list it as an official category with specific diagnostic criteria. All of this evidence suggests that chronic pain represents a special case, one that is different from standard biomedical disorders, such as diabetes or asthma, and also from official psychiatric diseases, such as depression. Rather, like chronic fatigue syndrome, chronic pain syndrome is a widely used clinical category without official sanction, an anomalous category, only partially legitimized as disease.

Chronic pain has an anomalous status in biomedicine largely because it is so baffling to clinicians and academic physicians. The pain is seldom adequately accounted for by physiological lesions; its course and outcome do not conform to any known biochemical or mechanical process. Although researchers have advanced competing neurological models, there is still no consensus on a unified conceptual framework for the diverse types of pain. In the absence of known physiological mechanisms, attention has turned to uncovering the social and psychological determinants of pain. Psychosocial factors are widely acknowledged as important influences in all chronic illness, and their role in chronic pain has received extensive study in diverse settings by researchers from various distinct traditions.

Psychologists and family therapists have studied the close association of chronic pain with social, psychiatric, and interpersonal problems. Psychologists, for example, have explored family patterns—emotional "enmeshment," rigidity, and overprotectiveness—which predispose individual members to chronic pain (Minuchin et al. 1978; Meissner 1974; Bokan et al. 1981). Some families may seize upon one member's pain symptom in order to detour conflict and maintain the household's emotional stability. Moreover, the family's response can strongly affect the disability and duration of chronic pain syndromes once established. Sympathy, increased attention, and nurturance positively reinforce such pain-related behaviors as use of medications and time spent in bed (Sternbach 1968; Fordyce 1976).

Psychiatric researchers have focused on the interrelations of depression, anxiety, and chronic pain disorders. Not only major depression but also less serious depressive symptoms and feelings of irritability or annoyance afflict patients with a wide range of pain complaints (Pilowsky and Spence 1976; Blumer and Heilbronn 1982; Pelz and Merskey 1982; Swanson 1984). Severe anxiety has been linked to specific pain disorders, including migraine headaches and temporomandibular joint disorders (examined in chaps. 2 and 5) (Henryk-Gutt and Rees 1973; Salter et al. 1983). However, critical readers should suspect these findings for two reasons. These studies report on patients already in treatment—a distinct (and distinctive) minority of all chronic pain sufferers (Chapman et al. 1979; Crooks, Rideout, and Browne 1984). Moreover, they beg the question of whether these psychological patterns help cause the pain or rather represent a common human response to the suffering of pain (see Merskey 1987).

These studies do, however, support the interpretation that chronic pain is a common idiom for communicating personal and interpersonal problems (Katon et al. 1982). Depression and anxiety, serious family tensions, conflicted work relationships—all conduce to the onset or exacerbation of chronic pain conditions and, in turn, may be worsened by chronic pain. Physical pain complaints therefore express painful relations and experiences. Psychiatrists and psychologists describe a range of meanings routinely expressed in complaints of chronic pain, from anger and loss to failure and fear (Engel 1959; Fordyce 1976; Melzack 1973; Sternbach 1974; Szasz 1959). At a societal level, Kleinman (1986) found that survivors of the devastating effects of China's Cultural Revolution articulated political disaffiliation in an idiom of complaint that made this crossover between bodily pain and existential pain.

Hilbert (1984), a sociologist, argues that chronic pain, because it is atypical or undiagnosable, escapes successful cultural construction. It defies the conventional meanings that patients try to place upon it. This renders pain a quintessentially anomic condition: no coherent system of values and beliefs emerges from the pain experience or survives its morally corrosive effects. The condition of chronic pain thus creates powerful double binds, explored by literary critic Elaine Scarry (1987). Pain is an inner experience, and even those closest to a patient cannot truly observe its progress or share in its suffering. Patients thus have no means to establish its validity as an "objective" part of the world for health professionals or society at large. Absolute private certainty to the sufferer, pain may become absolute public doubt to the observer. The upshot is often a pervasive distrust that undermines family as well as clinical relationships.

Pain can drive a wedge not only between the sufferers and those closest to them but also within pain sufferers themselves. The patient often experiences pain as an intrusive foreign agent: an unwelcome force producing great physical distress as well as moral and spiritual dilemmas. Others, however, see the patient as the agent, who somehow produces the pain as a response to social and psychological conditions. This approach implies that pain is at least partially willful, voluntary, and hence under the patient's control. This outsider's approach informs much of the psychological and psychosocial research on chronic pain (as described above) and stands at the basis of the ideology operative in certain treatment settings (see chap. 6). But it directly contradicts the immediate, unquestionable physical experience of most pain sufferers.

The National Academy of Sciences Institute of Medicine's report on *Pain and Disability* (Osterweis et al. 1987) concluded that there is no objective measure of pain—no "pain thermometer"—nor can there ever be one, because the experience of pain is inseparable from personal perception and social influence. Chronic pain thus challenges the central tenet of biomedical epistemology: namely, that there is objective knowledge, knowable apart from subjective experience (Kleinman 1988*b*; Good and Good 1981*b*; Gordon 1988). For this reason, the subject of chronic pain draws the researcher toward a cultural critique of biomedicine and of the societal values that are embedded deep within its concepts and practices.

WHY CHRONIC PAIN IS AN APPROPRIATE TOPIC FOR ANTHROPOLOGISTS

The theoretical resonance and practical salience of the study of chronic pain surely are reasons why anthropologists should be attracted to this subject. There are other reasons as well. Chronic pain is an important health problem that biomedicine has handled with astonishing lack of success. Medical care has more often than not compounded the suffering as a result of iatrogenic effects of powerful but dangerous surgical and pharmacological treatments and of costly and at times equally dangerous tests. Health professionals are widely viewed by chronic pain patients and their families as insensitive to the patient's needs and disaffirming of the illness experience, and—the ultimate irony—the relationships with health professionals are seen as untherapeutic (see Corbett 1986). By pointing to a source of systematic failure in the health-care system, chronic pain focuses the gaze of the anthropologist on serious weaknesses in the way health professionals are trained and health care is "delivered" in the United States. The ambiguity of chronic pain opens for analysis a site in American medicine where the relations of power and professional knowledge and the potential for exploitation residing in power relations are unusually visible.

Professional biomedical care is not the only culprit. Chronic pain is addressed, often with equally little success, by alternative professional practices, folk healing, and self-care as well. Chronic pain patients and their families are dissatisfied, often vehemently so, with the health-care system, every component of which has failed them. Thus, the study of chronic pain leads the researcher to examine a dimension of American medicine that is as much a part of the problem as the solution, offering anthropologists the occasion for critical analysis. Chronic pain not only exposes basic contradictions of medical ideology and care to analysis but also suggests the importance of more systematic criticism of efforts to contain and manage fundamental aspects of human suffering through technical mastery and instrumental rationality.

Anthropological concern with chronic pain arises also from the impressive social problems it indexes: the noxious effects of environmental hazards and power structures in the workplace (Susser 1988), the crisis in the disability and welfare system, the negative consequences of medicalization, and the growth of a "market" for pain products, pain professionals, and pain institutes. We are witnessing the political economic transformation of pain and its treatment—a small but particularly telling feature in the immense transformation of the American health-care enterprise in our times. Medical anthropologists interested in political economy research (see Morgan 1987 for a review) will thus find the potential here for important investigations.

Even more, however, the study of chronic pain seems appropriate to the growing interest in medical anthropology in embodied experience (e.g., Csordas 1990). Anthropologists concerned with the anthropology of everyday experience and the embodiment of cultural categories of distress are drawn to pain in order to understand how the bodily experience itself is influenced by meanings, relationships, and institutions (Kleinman 1988a; Devisch 1983; Csordas 1990; Good and Good 1981b; Kaufman 1988). These medical and psychological anthropologists are frustrated with the "business as usual" examination of suffering which subsumes personal experience within local cultural categories. They recognize that human conditions such as pain are not adequately appreciated if the analysis begins and ends with the exploration of linguistic terms and cultural taxonomies. Pain itself poses an obdurate resistance to cultural categories. It is an experience that simply cannot be avoided, an experience that sets limits to the meanings given it by cultural beliefs, discourses, or practices. Something is at stake, frequently desperately so, in the lives of pain patients. Pain can be a massive threat to the legitimacy of the everyday world. Viewed in these terms, the anthropological study of chronic pain addresses the sources, varieties, and consequences of human suffering.

MONISTIC PAIN/DUALISTIC MEDICINE

Pain, as Scarry (1985) writes, defies language. It occurs on that fundamental level of bodily experience which language encounters, attempts to express, and then fails to encompass. Perhaps more than other somatic experiences, pain resists symbolization. Language and categories may rework and re-shape pain, but they cannot remove or avoid it. Nonetheless, while pain appears at one moment as an unmediated and unmistakable fact, the next moment it seems produced by a dialectic interaction of biological and social processes (see Buytendijk 1974). The experience of chronic pain includes much more than raw physical sensation: pain creates problems of control and meaning-making. It demands enormous energy in the search for relief (see Kotarba 1983; Fagerhaugh and Strauss 1977; Baszanger 1989). These activities incorporate the contradictions of the health-care system into the life world of sufferers and their families. These personal and social responses to pain thus remake the everyday worlds of patients and their families.

Most social scientists studying chronic pain recognize the gap between lay worlds of pain and the world of pain constituted in health-care settings (e.g., Kotarba 1983; Murphy 1987; Zola 1982). The core conflicts between pain patients and health professionals involve many factors—frustration on both sides over the inadequacy of therapeutic interventions, distrust over the assessment of pain and its implications for disability determinations, and disagreement over the influence of voluntary control over symptoms and on the question of accountability. Yet one conflict is so fundamental it has preoccupied social science students of pain. However complicated to articulate and difficult to interpret, the patient's experience of pain is lived as a whole. Perception, experience, and coping run into each other and are lived as a unified experience.[2] When reconstituted as a medical problem, however, that experience is fragmented into a series of dichotomies that represent the deep cultural logic of biomedicine. Physiological, psychological; body, soul; mind, body; subjective, objective; real, unreal; natural, artificial—these dichotomies, so deeply rooted in the Western world and its profession of medicine, are at the heart of the struggle between chronic pain patients and their care givers over the definition of the problem and the search for effective treatment.

In Gordon's analysis (1988) of a series of "tenacious assumptions in West-ern medicine," the idea of the autonomy of nature is central. In Western medicine, nature (biology to practitioners) is opposed to spirit; it is auton-omous from human consciousness (subjective experience); each of its parts is atomistic, independent from the whole; and it "stands not only in-dependent from culture but prior to it" (Gordon 1988:27). Furthermore, nature is a realm separate from morality and society (Taylor 1989). Nature, so isolated, is regarded as universal. It is not dependent upon the param-eters of space and time. Nature—biology—is the basis for truth itself. To know nature is to see it: in the body, in the test tube, under the microscope (Good and Good 1989). The order of nature is rational, and human ration-ality provides the means for explaining natural phenomena. (And, we might add, rationality is usually self-defined as the expert's set of thoughts.)

Gordon (1988) identifies a second category of tenacious assumptions in Western-rooted biomedicine. The individual is a sovereign being, a distinct unit, prior to society and culture, and *autonomous* from them (see Taylor 1985). The knower, the subject of knowledge, is the rational individual whose cognitive states reflect an image of the natural world. The human actor is an individual agent who uses instrumental reason to accomplish goals in the everyday world. Individual orientation is as much part of biomedicine as it is part of Western culture. Sickness is resident in the individual, in individual physiology, and diagnosis and therapy focus exclusive gaze upon the individual body. Suffering is the private response of the subject, and as long as that subject is competent, the moral responsibility of the physician is limited to the individual sufferer.

Now think what egregious influence these values exert on medical practice with patients suffering chronic pain or other chronic illness (see Kleinman 1988*a*, 1988*b*). The experience of chronic pain is fundamentally intersubjective. Chronic pain profoundly affects the lives of the family, intimate friends, co-workers, and even at times the care giver, and such persons in turn shape the experiential world of the sufferer. To regard pain as the experience of an individual, as it is regarded in standard biomedical practice, is so inadequate as to virtually assure inaccurate diagnosis and unsuccessful treatment. Yet this is only the tip of the iceberg.

For the biomedical researcher, pain is the result of change in "material" structures: sensory receptors, afferent neuronal relays, way stations in spinal-cord, mid-brain, or higher cortical modulating systems. The paradigm of investigation—on either the molecular or physiological level—is reductionistic. It reduces the experience of pain to etiological "mechanisms": biological processes that are measured in "objective," quantitative terms, most valid when most material. Thus, tissue pathology is more valid than electro-physiological pathology. But this value formulation directly eschews what is most essential to the experience of pain—namely, the relationship between neurobiological and social psychological processes.

Complex processes transform painful relationships and pained feelings into chest pain and, vice versa, transform chest pain into a painful world. These "sociosomatic" processes, processes that inscribe history and social relations onto the body, simply cannot be reduced to biological terminology without distorting in the most fundamental way what pain or, for that matter, experience per se is about.

Biological reductionism also fails to illuminate what constitutes chronicity and disability. From the perspective of biomedical research and orthodox clinical practice, chronic illnesses have a "natural course," which is in essence the unfolding of a predetermined plan of development within the diathesis, the disease as an elemental, natural phenomenon. Disability, in the same discourse, is the impairment that results from the "natural course" of the disorder. Now these assumptions are curiously at odds with the everyday world of pain patients.

For when the latter, unable to continue working, encounter the disability system, they quickly learn that disability is an administrative category established by the SSA based upon congressional regulations (Osterweis et al. 1987). In this sense, disability is a political category to a much greater extent than it is a biological one (Stone 1984; cf. Warner 1985). Because of the often powerful influence of unemployment, perceived quality of work and work relationships, family, ecology, and mood on the outcome of pain, chronicity cannot be construed as the "natural course" of a particular pathological condition (see McQueen and Siegrist 1982; Turner and Noh 1988; Egan and Katon 1987).

Individuals with the same pathology may develop vastly different disabilities because pain has different meanings for their lives (Lipowski 1969; McHugh and Vallis 1986). The site of the pathology may be precisely the same, yet the course is likely to be quite different, depending on the meaning of the pain, the life world of the sick person, and his or her relationship to family, health-care and disability systems, and the resources available to treat pain. The case studies in this volume vividly demonstrate that inasmuch as pain is always lived as a particular kind of human experience, there can be no "natural course" of a chronic pain syndrome.

Psychological studies claim to challenge this type of biological reductionism. Instead of grounding pain in the objective condition of the body, they regard pain as produced or maintained according to known psychological principles. This psychological literature, however, often reproduces the same conventional categories underlying the medical approach. By focusing exclusively on the psychological sources of pain, such studies scrupulously respect the categorical distinction between body and mind. The medical literature privileges objective somatic processes, and it enshrines them as the agent that produces pain. The psychological literature takes the opposite position: it imputes agency to the subjective mind (as affected by specific behavioral contingencies and family dynamics); these mindful processes then produce physical pain. The Cartesian dichotomy remains unquestioned. Both traditions tend to ignore how a person's immediate experience of pain unites its bodily, psychological, and social origins (see Brodwin and Kleinman 1987).

Much psychological research begins with the notion of "secondary gains" and the behaviorist principles of operant conditioning. This model predicts that the rewards provided by a patient's environment will act as the prime incentive for chronic pain disorders. For example, the responses of family members can significantly affect the disability caused by chronic pain. Sympathy, increased attention, and nurturance may reinforce pain behaviors (Sternbach 1968; Fordyce 1976). Hudgens (1979) lists other secondary gains secured by chronic pain: controlling others, justifying dependency, earning rest, avoiding sex, gaining attention, punishing others, controlling anger, and avoiding close relationships. These secondary gains may have destructive effects, and Menges (1981) describes the manipulative "pain games" of patients who use their symptoms to dominate other family members or escape responsibilities.

Minuchin et al. (1978) shifts the psychological focus from individual behavior to family systems. He examines how "psychosomatic families" seize upon a child's physical symptom in order to detour conflict and maintain the family's stability. When negative feelings remain unexpressed, focusing on the chronic pain in a vulnerable family member, especially a child, is less threatening than revealing an emotional problem (Meissner 1974; Liebman et al. 1976; Hughes and Zimin 1978).[3]

In addition to these behaviorist and psychodynamic studies, psychologists have investigated how social learning and modeling influence chronic pain. Pain patients have often witnessed similar suffering among their kin; chronic pain is more common among family members of such patients than among families of persons with other chronic illnesses (Violon and Giurgea 1984). The influence of available family models may even be symptom specific. Headache patients have a disproportionate number of family members who also suffer from headaches (Turkat et al. 1984). The rate of abdominal pain in parents of children with chronic abdominal pain is six times higher than in a control group (Apley 1975). Pain patients may thus have "familial pain models" that influence the onset of chronic pain as well as its disability (Edwards et al. 1985).

The dichotomy between mind and body upheld by both medical and psychological research is invalid and unavailing. Yet it is the viewpoint of many practitioners, most researchers, and not a few patients. Patients are mortified and angered to find their experience discredited as "not real" or "functional" pain (see Jackson, chap. 6). Families must struggle to empathize with the effects of pain on a loved one, while at the same time they are told the pain is "a psychological, not a medical, problem." Practitioners with "psychosomatic" orientation must continually remind themselves that biological and social psychological processes interrelate, in spite of reading research literature that overwhelmingly decries the significance of such interrelationships and of encountering clinical colleagues who denigrate a "biopsychosocial" viewpoint as "soft" and quaintly unbiomedical.

Historical and psychiatric evidence attests to the widespread adoption of a psychological idiom of distress by the middle class in Europe and North America. Clinicians today rarely encounter the classic hysteria and conversion symptoms of late nineteenth-century Vienna. But have well-educated "psychologically-minded" individuals abandoned a somatic idiom entirely? Does the somatic presentation of psychological and social distress appear only in nonwhite ethnic groups and lower social classes, social groups that lie outside the mainstream of the therapeutic state (Leff 1981)?

One of the chief findings presented in this book is a resounding no to both questions. The case studies portray middle-class white Americans who readily and profoundly exploit physical symptoms to communicate personal distress. For many of us, somatization—an idiom of physically painful signs and symptoms—has become stabilized alongside the reigning discourse of emotions and inner feelings.[4] The sufferers of chronic pain, in particular, have elaborated these two parallel and interacting languages in their talk about symptoms and their search for relief. The actual prevalence of classic hysterical and conversion symptoms may have decreased. However, these two cultural languages—one indexing the body and the other indexing the self and its social transactions—continue to inform our understanding of chronic pain and chronic illness generally.

That so many individuals have recourse to these complementary discourses proves the inadequacy of the crude Cartesian mind-body dualism described above. This book focuses on both a class of patients and a few unique individuals who communicate their distress simultaneously through symptoms and words. It thereby suggests how modern Americans attempt to transcend the dichotomy of thought and sensation which is inscribed in everyday language, medical jargon, and treatment settings. They do not transcend it entirely, as the following pages make clear through the many examples of failed self-understanding, miscommunication within families, and frustrating impasses between patients and clinicians. But for the discerning reader (and sensitive clinician), the expression of suffering through both words *and* physical symptoms constitutes an understandable and familiar human language.

PAIN AND THE NATURE OF HUMAN SUFFERING

In his searching account of the massive brutality and day-to-day inhumanity suffered by the frontline soldier in World War II, Robert Fussel (1989), himself a combat veteran of that grisly "conventional" war, writes of soldiers having to endure the unendurable—horrible wounds, constant fear, the likelihood of death at any moment—without the sense of control or coherence or the possibility of transcendence. That is a description of a particular form of suffering. Primo Levi (1961) describes those who succumbed or survived the systemization of murder at Auschwitz; Haing Ngor (1987) recounts the experience of those who underwent the mind-numbing horrors of the Cambodian genocide; Nien Cheng (1986) speaks for the victims of China's Cultural Revolution; Veena Das (1989) describes the misery of victims of Bhopal and of the Hindu riots against Sikhs after the assassination of Indira Gandhi. The list of contemporary forms of suffering is despairingly long. Its scope extends from the havoc of war and revolution and other man-made or "natural" disasters to routinization of suffering brought about by dehumanizing poverty, systematic discrimination, community-wide drug or alcohol abuse and their violent sequelae, or the even more intimate oppression in workplace or family. Looking back over the epochs in the historical record and across the boundaries of greatly different societies, we see so many sources of suffering—plagues, famines, slavery, astonishingly high rates of child and maternal mortality and of child and adult abuse, to name a few of the more notorious—that it would seem that suffering is a defining characteristic of the human condition.

Certainly death, pain, disfigurement, impairment of functioning, humiliating symptoms, the fear of uncertain outcome, the loss of capacity and relationships, and all the other ways that *illness* can assault the person and the group figure as both common and powerful forms of suffering. Much of "traditional" medical care across epochs and societies has centered on the experience of suffering. What do patients most appreciate in the medical care they receive? Arguably, it is the attention that care givers devote to the experience of menacing symptoms and grave loss as much as the technical interventions that improve outcome. *Pain* is often used as a graphic illustration of the suffering caused by illness, of the body or of the mind. Therefore, to relieve pain is to alleviate suffering. When therapy fails, however, or even when it succeeds, the offer of personal and family support in face of the burdens of illness, bearing witness to the moral experience of suffering, providing suffering with a coherent meaning, and preparing for a socially appropriate death and for religious transcendence are universal features of societal responses to suffering.

Suffering is not just expressed but constituted through lay and expert discourses on its sources and consequences. The medieval quest for religious transcendence shaped the responses of whole societies as well as families and individuals to the Black Death. The suffering caused by that plague thus differs dramatically from the societal response to the pain and death from AIDS in our times (Gottfried 1984; Sontag 1989).[5] What is so impressive about current forms of suffering is the relative weakening in the modern era of moral and religious vocabularies, both in collective representations and the language of experts. In their place we see the proliferation of rational-technical professional argots that express and constitute suffering in physiological, public health, clinical, psychological, and policy terms. These secular discourses accomplish what Max Weber predicted early in this century they might achieve: namely, to replace the "looser," ad hoc, fuzzier talk about sentiment and tradition—for example, talk of yearning, misery, aspirations, and transcendence—with the much more systematic, routinized, quantified talk about biomedical and psychiatric and legal and policy issues. The transformation of language is notable, even within the social sciences, for leaving out the human spirit and the sacred. In the contemporary discourses on pain or other forms of suffering—expert and popular—the idea of suffering has been attenuated, sometimes trivialized, and at times expunged altogether, although it may remain resonant in the personal and family encounter with suffering. Neither in the biomedical research literature nor in the pain clinic does the *suffering* of pain patients and their intimate social circles receive much attention as such, that is, as a moral burden or a defining existential experience. Pain as human suffering in the dominant institutions that deal with it in our times is a question of therapeutic *means*—analgesia, surgical procedures, rehabilitation, psychotherapy—not of human (or suprahuman) *ends*.

The upshot is that the intricate experience as much as the straightforward treatments of pain are culturally embedded. Moreover, the symbolic processes that interrelate body and self with meanings and relationships change as part of wider societal and cultural transformations (Kleinman 1986). Pain and suffering have thus also changed over time. Charting the causes, features, and implications of this astonishing transformation in the human condition in the West and contrasting it with other societies and other times should be what distinguishes the anthropology of pain from the biology and psychology of pain.

This approach suggests the importance of placing the study of human suffering in a broader historical and civilizational frame. What have been the primary modalities of conceiving, shaping, and responding to suffering across history and society? And how have European and North American traditions compared with those of other civilizations? Is there an "experiential transition" discernible through history, one that parallels the more widely noted demographic and epidemiological transitions?[6] If it exists, does that transition involve similar dimensions of change? Does it vary for different societies and for different groups within societies? What are the consequences of this hypothesized "experiential transition" for pain patients, families, and health professionals in our own society? These are large questions that future studies in the anthropology of pain might profitably address.

OVERVIEW OF THE VOLUME

For the purpose of this edited volume, we have set ourselves a more modest agenda. We have developed a set of studies of *experiences of chronic pain*, in the context of American culture and society, which highlight the daily effects of pain, its place in the biography of the pain sufferer, its trajectory through the family and workplace, its treatment, and the effects of cultural and social forces upon each element of the pain experience. Taken together, these studies establish the domain of suffering inhabited by pain patients. They reveal the intimate and shared meanings pain holds for an individual, a family, or care givers, meanings that color patients' experience of the everyday world.

We have attempted to write an *ethnography of experience* of persons afflicted by chronic pain. Like all ethnographies, this volume explores the crucial categories that exert a strong but unseen effect on these people's lives: How does pain feel? What is at stake for the sick person and family? What is learned from the encounter with pain by those who undergo it and those who provide care? How is the meaning of pain created, expressed, and negotiated? How are meanings reflected or constituted in stories people tell? What is the relation between such narratives and lived experience? And how do the meanings of pain and suffering emerge from, and then reciprocally influence, particular worlds of pain? If the book clarifies this iterative process of experience lived under bodily constraint, of the making of painful meanings, and of the meanings of painful worlds, if we illustrate that iterative, dialectical process with enough convincing detail, it will have succeeded.

The contributors bring to this book differing questions of social theory, different anthropological preoccupations, even different investigations with different samples of pain patients. Yet we all share participation, at one time or another, in the Harvard Program in Medical Anthropology's "Friday Morning Seminar." That weekly seminar, supported with funds from a training grant from the National Institutes of Mental Health,[7] has both a scholarly and a practical mission. It reviews the methodological developments and conceptual controversies in anthropological studies of health and health care; it also discusses the relevance of these for practical questions confronting patients, clinicians, and policymakers. Since its inception, the seminar has placed great emphasis on studies of the experienced worlds of patients and healers and on the refashioning of research methodologies, especially interpretive ones, to pursue with greater validity our understanding of body-self processes, illness narratives, and the changing social contexts within which illness and clinical practice are enacted.

The Seminar's colloquy is the backdrop for the research projects reported in this volume. These include a study of chronic pain supported by the National Science Foundation, a study of jaw, neck, and back pain, and an NIMH-funded ethnography of a single residential pain clinic. The NSF-supported study, "The Ethnography of Chronic Somatization,"[8] carried out by the editors of this volume, investigated four aspects of chronic pain in working Americans: the experience and meaning of their symptoms, the history of illness and loss in their families, the range of their associated emotional problems, and their social disabilities and work adaptations. Intensive interviews were carried out with thirty-eight patients over two years. The sample differed from many such studies in that participants were employed and working at the time they entered the study. Chapters 3, 4, and 7 depict participants in this study.[9] The study of sufferers of jaw, neck, and back pain was carried out by Linda Garro, Karen Stevenson, and Byron Good. Lengthy interviews were conducted with forty persons, thirty-two of whom suffered jaw joint pain or dysfunction, drawn from volunteers from several chronic illness support groups. Chapters 2 and 5 provide in-depth accounts of several of these pain sufferers. Finally, chapter 6 reports the results of an ethnographic investigation of a well-known chronic-pain treatment center on the East Coast. This two-year study, conducted by Jean Jackson, was supported by a grant from the NIMH.[10]

The anthropology of experience is the shared conceptual thread uniting these chapters; it is the identifying signature that emerges from the authors' participation in the Harvard seminar. The chapters attempt (1) to provide an authentic representation of the experiences sufferers have been willing to share with us, and (2) to draw generalizations from the analysis of these "microscopic" experiential accounts, or (3) to examine that experience as refigured in diverse treatment contexts.

Chapter 2, by Byron Good, provides a phenomenological analysis of the complex array of pains of a single young man, who ascribes his pain to an underlying temporomandibular joint disorder. The analysis suggests that studies of the pain experience not only should attend to direct reports of experience but might begin with investigation of the experienced world, the "life world." Drawing on Alfred Schutz (a German-American philosopher and sociologist) and Elaine Scarry's volume on pain (1985), the chapter explores the perceptual dimensions through which this young man's life world is constituted, the radical reshaping of that world under the influence of enduring pain, and the constant threat of dissolution of that achieved world for the chronic pain sufferer. In addition, the chapter provides an analysis of the young man's "origin myth," or narrative of the onset and foundation of the pain. A close reading of the text indicates that two conflicting narratives, one of psychological origins and one of physiological sources of the pain, are juxtaposed. But since neither have provided final grounds for therapeutic efficacy, neither provides a final reading of the experience.

Mary-Jo DelVecchio Good, in chapter 3, examines the relationship of work and chronic pain among two women who are part of a special category of pain patients to which many of those who participated in these studies belonged. These are professional women who continue actively working in spite of chronic pain, which many of them experience daily. Unlike pain patients who have been the focus of most research—those who because of chronic pain are unemployed or on the disability rolls—for these two women, work is a haven from pain. Work provides a meaningful way of being-in-the-world, in spite of histories replete with losses, menace, dissatisfaction, and disappointments in their personal and family lives. Work is both a mode of self-realization and an occasion for the purposive control over the intrusiveness of pain, physical and psychological, into the day-to-day world. Through work, these women actively engage the world, attending to their professional activities and demands as opposed to their bodies in pain. This chapter thus suggests a reinterpretation of much of the literature on gender, work, and pain.

In chapter 4, Paul Brodwin depicts a woman whose pain, while neither disabling nor particularly intense, has yet come to dominate her entire life. This young woman relies almost exclusively on physical symptoms for emotional communication with her family and friends. Her pain thus functions like a language, and it speaks with an authenticity and power that her verbal messages often lack. The particular symptoms from which she suffers have varied considerably over time. But throughout her life, she has made use of pain symptoms either to influence her treatment by those around her or to try to resolve her particular personal dilemma: establishing an independent identity in a constraining and traditional social milieu.

The role of chronic pain sufferer has become a performance that she cannot (or does not want to) end. But the case has a twist, a lived irony, for Brodwin shows that this intelligent woman knows what she is doing: she is aware of the performance, which her pain occasions, how it protests against an alienating and subservient role, and how it substitutes for more direct life changes. Brodwin thus recommends the metaphor of performance for the study of chronic pain. This approach assumes that not only do patients suffer from their pain but they employ it in different ways and to different ends in the various life-roles they play. The performative approach also highlights the dramaturgic, at times theatrical, transactions between chronic pain patients and their families and co-workers. By examining these performances over time, it suggests why they may persist with such strength.

Linda Garro demonstrates in chapter 5 that patients with the confusing conditions of temporomandibular joint pain and cranial injury encounter an ontological assault, a threat to their life plan and self identity. These patients' stories of sickness center on the search for effective treatment, a quest that assumes form in the very gap between biomedicine's technical criteria for treatment and the popular culture's criteria for evaluating alternative therapies. This conceptual gap, as we have already seen, reflects the dichotomies between body and pain and mind and pain. Garro's research illustrates how a common cognitive form, a prototypical narrative structure, and the process of reconstructing the past and constructing the present and future underlie these stories of pain.

Jean Jackson portrays, in chapter 6, a chronic pain unit which employs a unique and, to some patients, quite troubling, psychosomatic discourse. This discourse makes problematic whether pain is "real" and whether one is accountable for careers of pain and for the stigma pain causes. It throws into doubt fundamental aspects of patients' experience, supposedly in order to insert a thin therapeutic wedge into illness careers that resonate hostility, self-defeat, and previous treatment failure. Are the patients, whom Jackson shows to be confused by the shifting terms of the treatment ideology, supposed to be confused, to become hostile to the medical establishment? Do they get better? Is their improvement because of, or in spite of, the therapeutic ideology?

This pain center, Jackson's ethnography shows us, mystifies patients about pain, thus reflecting and reproducing the mystification of pain in the wider society. Is this seemingly paradoxical treatment effective? While few patients appear to see themselves as significantly improved, much less converted to the clinic's assumptive world, Jackson does not state that the program is unsuccessful. Rather, her chapter lays the groundwork for a more complex appreciation of the meaning of transformation of symptoms and illness behavior. Jackson's work reassesses the conflict between the patients' world of pain and suffering and its clinical and biomedical reformulation, suggesting that this clash of unequal perspectives may actually have a therapeutic effect.

Finally, Arthur Kleinman, in chapter 7, provides analyses of two cases of chronic pain sufferers from the NSF study and reflections on his previous research in China to explore the emergence of the lived flow of pain experience in local moral worlds. Kleinman argues that pain is experienced as a form of "resistance" in two senses of the word. Pain confronts the sufferer, limits plans and practical activities, resists efforts to avoid or overcome it, and thus provokes suffering. Pain also serves as a medium for resistance in the more recent analytic sense of the word: as a means for resisting oppressive social relationships. Pain provides the occasion and a language for resisting forms of domination present in family relations, in political and economic structures, and in the often alienating activities of medical diagnosis and treatment. At times it enables the sufferer to resist such oppressive structures more eloquently than any available discourse. Yet, Kleinman argues, pain is often ineffective as a form of resistance. Moreover, its analysis in these terms often gives primacy to coherent meanings and to social science accounts, thus appropriating the experience of that for which there are no words. Configured as suffering, pain evokes intractable existential, moral, and spiritual questions and forms of experience that are as vulnerable to dehumanizing social scientific accounts as to the biomedical. This final observation describes the context in which anthropologists carry out such studies and reaffirms the importance of faithful attention to the lived experience of those with whom we work.

In sum, the chapters of this collection provide an anthropological contribution to the analysis of chronic pain in American culture. All assume the profound importance of regnant cultural dichotomies, referred to earlier, in shaping both professional and popular discourse about pain. These cultural categories are "social facts," aspects of the real world—the culturally constituted behavioral environment, as Hallowell (1955) called it—which have tremendous force in shaping experience and social institutions, but which also reflect the institutions in which they are embedded. They influence modes of reasoning about pain, its sources and treatment, and society's responsibility for its sufferers. They thus contribute, subtly and yet with force, to the building of personal perception and experience. They are embedded in everyday discourse and clinical communications, institutionalized in therapeutic and compensation practices. Cultural categories are simultaneously intimate and alien, at once pain's dancer and its dance.

This volume, however, does not offer primarily a symbolic or semiotic analysis of American cultural categories and the presuppositions that frame American medicine. Instead, these essays present detailed accounts of individual lives or treatment settings and analyze how cultural categories interact with social situations and psychological constraints to transform the experience and the lives of sufferers. They demonstrate the great variation of the incorporation of public meanings into the personal lives of those afflicted with pain. They provide self-conscious methodological approaches to the analysis of such lives, drawing in particular from phenomenology, narrative analysis, practice theory, and studies of everyday forms of resistance. And they recommend directions for the cross-cultural study of one critical mode of human experience and human suffering.

NOTES

1. Melzack (1989), for example, who draws on the condition of phantom limb pain to underpin his theory of the "neurosignatures" that emerge from the brain-self's "neuromatrix." For Melzack, the neuromatrix comprises central nervous system constraints on experience that occur even independent of peripheral sensory signals.

2. See Michael Oakeshott (1985 [1933]) on the unifying quality of worlds of experience, and William James (1981) and Henri Bergson (1960) on the lived flow of experience.

3. Bokan et al. (1981) use the term "tertiary gain" to identify social sources that maintain chronic pain behavior owing to "gains" received by family members, intimate others, even the practitioner.

4. This finding is in line with the contributions of Mechanic and his collaborators (1972) who disclose that, contrary to a psychoanalytic account of somatization, subjects who score high in scales of somatic symptoms also score high on scales of psychological complaints.

5. But compare Sontag's (1989) cultural critique of AIDS as suffering in our times to the personal accounts of AIDS sufferers—e.g., Dreuilhe (1988)—to see how even a sensitive writer, following contemporary postmodernist preoccupations, is led away from the meaning of suffering as experience to the meaning of suffering as cultural metaphor.

6. Current public health research on the "health transition" in developing societies focuses largely on the reduction of infant mortality and rates of infectious diseases and the emergence of new forms and sources of morbidity, in particular chronic diseases. However, it does not link these trends to the transformation of illness experience. Researchers would do well to address the question of whether the demographic and health transitions will be accompanied by a weakening and even abandonment of a language of suffering and its replacement with the technical language of biomedicine and public health.

7. The Training Program in Clinically Relevant Medical Anthropology is sup-

ported by NIMH research training grant MH 18006. Arthur Kleinman and Byron Good are codirectors of the training grant.

8. NSF Grant No. 83-09816, Principal Investigator Arthur Kleinman.

9. Additional case studies drawn from this group are analyzed in chaps. 3, 4, 5, and 11 of Kleinman's *The Illness Narratives* (1988), which might be read as a companion volume to this one.

10. NIMH Research Grant No. MH 41787, Principal Investigator Jean Jackson.

REFERENCES CITED

Abad, V., and E. Boyce
  1979   Issues in psychiatric evaluations of Puerto Ricans: A sociocultural perspective. *Journal of Operational Psychiatry* 10:28–39.
Agnew, D., and H. Merskey
  1976   Words of chronic pain. *Pain* 2:73–81.
Alexander, L.
  1982   Illness maintenance and the new American sick role. In *Clinically applied anthropology*, N. Chrisman and T. Maretzki, eds., 352–367. Dordrecht, Holland: D. Reidel Publishing Co.
Anderson, L., and L. Rehm
  1984   The relationship between strategies of coping and perception of pain in three chronic pain groups. *Journal of Clinical Psychology* 40:1170–1177.
Apley, J.
  1975   *The child with abdominal pain.* Oxford: Blackwell Press.
Bailey, C., and P. Davidson
  1976   The language of pain: Intensity. *Pain* 2:319–324.
Barsky, A.
  1979   Patients who amplify bodily sensation. *Annals of Internal Medicine* 91:63–70.
Baszanger, I.
  1989   Pain: Its experience and treatments. *Social Science and Medicine* 29(3): 425–434.
Bergson, H.
  1960   *Time and free will: An essay on the immediate data of consciousness.* New York: Harper & Brothers.
Berkowitz, M.
  1987   Economic issues and the cost of disability. In *Pain and disability: Clinical, behavioral, and public policy perspectives*, M. Osterweis et al., eds., 87–100. Washington, D.C.: National Academy Press.
Block, A., E. Kremer, and M. Gaylor
  1980   Behavioral treatment of chronic pain: Variables affecting treatment efficacy. *Pain* 8:367–375.
Blumer, D., and M. Heilbronn
  1982   Chronic pain as a variant of depressive disease: The pain prone disorder. *Journal of Nervous and Mental Disease* 170:381–394.
Bokan, J., R. Ries, and W. Katon
  1981   Tertiary gain and chronic pain. *Pain* 10:331–335.

Bowen, M.
  1978   *Family therapy in clinical practice.* New York: Jason Aronson.
Brena, S., S. Chapman, P. Stegall, and S. Chayette
  1979   Chronic pain states: Their relationship to impairment and disability. *Archives of Physical Medicine and Rehabilitation* 60:387–389.
Brihaye, J., F. Loew, and H. Pia
  1987   *Pain: A medical and anthropological challenge.* Acta Neurochirurgica Supplementum 38. New York: Springer-Verlag.
Brodwin, P., and A. Kleinman
  1987   The social meanings of chronic pain. In *Handbook of chronic pain management*, G. Burrows, D. Elton, and G. Stanley, eds., 109–119. Amsterdam: Elsevier Scientific Publishers.
Buytendijk, F. J. J.
  1974   *Prolegomena to an anthropological physiology.* Pittsburgh: Duquesne University Press.
Carron, H., D. DeGood, and R. Tait
  1985   A comparison of low back pain patients in the United States and New Zealand: Psychological and economic factors affecting severity of disability. *Pain* 21:77–89.
Cassell, E.
  1982   The nature of suffering and the goals of medicine. *New England Journal of Medicine* 306:639–645.
Catchlove, R., and K. Cohen
  1982   Effects of a directive return to work approach in the treatment of workmen's compensation patients with chronic pain. *Pain* 14:181–191.
Chapman, S., S. Brena, and L. Bradford
  1981   Treatment outcome in a chronic pain rehabilitation program. *Pain* 11:255–268.
Chapman, S., A. Sola, and J. Bonica
  1979   Illness behavior and depression compared in pain center and private practice patients. *Pain* 6:1–7.
Cheng, N.
  1986   *Life and death in Shanghai.* New York: Grove Press.
Cleveland, M.
  1979   Family adaptation to the traumatic spinal cord injury of a son or daughter. *Social Work and Health Care* 4:459–471.
Corbett, K. K.
  1986   Adding insult to injury: Cultural dimensions of frustration in the management of chronic back pain. Ph.D. diss., joint doctoral program in medical anthropology, University of California, Berkeley and San Francisco.
Craig, K., and M. Wyckoff
  1987   Cultural factors in chronic pain management. In *Handbook of chronic pain management*, G. Burrows et al., eds., 99–108. Amsterdam: Elsevier Scientific Publishers.
Crooks, J., E. Rideout, and G. Browne
  1984   The prevalence of pain complaints in a general population. *Pain* 18:299–314.

Csordas, T.
1983   The rhetoric of transformation in ritual healing. *Culture, Medicine and Psychiatry* 7:333–375.
1990   Embodiment as a paradigm for anthropology. *Ethos* 18:5–47.

Das, V.
1989   What is health? Paper presented at "Health Transition Seminar," Center for Population Studies, Harvard University, May 1989.

Devisch, R.
1983   Eaten up with pain: A semantic-anthropological view of epigastric complaints. Paper prepared for XIth International Congress of Anthropological and Ethnological Sciences, Quebec City, IS-19, August 1983.

Dreuilhe, E.
1988   *Mortal embrace: Living with AIDS.* New York: Hill and Wang.

Dworkin, R., D. Handlin, D. Richlin, L. Brand, and C. Vanunucci
1985   Unraveling the effects of compensation, litigation, and employment on treatment response in chronic pain. *Pain* 23:49–59.

Ebigbo, P. O.
1982   Development of a culture specific (Nigerian) screening scale of somatic complaints. *Culture, Medicine and Psychiatry* 6:29–44.

Edwards, P., Z. Zeichner, A. Kuczmierczyk, and J. Boczkowski
1985   Familial pain models: The relationship between family history of pain and current pain experience. *Pain* 21:379–384.

Egan, K., and W. Katon
1987   Responses to illness and health in chronic pain patients and healthy adults. *Psychosomatic Medicine* 49:470–481.

Engel, G.
1959   Psychogenic pain and the pain prone patient. *American Journal of Medicine* 26:899–918.

Fabrega, H., and S. Tyma
1976a   Culture, language, and the shaping of illness: An illustration based on pain. *Journal of Psychosomatic Research* 20:323–337.
1976b   Language and cultural influence in the description of pain. *British Journal of Medical Psychology* 49:349–371.

Fagerhaugh, S. Y., and A. Strauss
1977   *Politics of pain management: Staff-patient interaction.* New York: Addison-Wesley Publishing Co.

Fernandez, J.
1972   Persuasions and performances: Of the beast in every body . . . and the metaphors of everyman. *Daedalus* 101(1) Winter: 39–60.
1974   The mission of metaphor in expressive culture. *Current Anthropology* 15: 119–145.

Fordyce, W.
1976   *Behavioral methods for chronic pain and illness.* St. Louis, Mo.: Mosby Press.

Framo, J.
1970   Symptoms from a family transactional viewpoint. In *Family therapy in transition*, N. Ackerman, J. Lieb, and J. Pearce, eds. Boston: Little, Brown & Co.

Frankenberg, R.
    1986   Sickness as cultural performance: Drama, trajectory, and pilgrimage root metaphors and the making social of disease. *International Journal of Health Services* 16(4): 603–626.
Fussel, R.
    1989   The real war, 1939–1945. *Atlantic Monthly*, August 1989:32–40.
Goffman, E.
    1959   *The presentation of self in everyday life.* New York: Doubleday Anchor Books.
Good, B., and M. J. Good
    1981a   The meaning of symptoms: A cultural hermeneutic model for clinical practice. In *The relevance of social science for medicine*, L. Eisenberg and A. Kleinman, eds., 166–196. Dordrecht, Holland: D. Reidel Publishing Co.
    1981b   The semantics of medical discourse. In *Sciences and cultures: Sociology of the sciences*, vol. 5, E. Mendelsohn and Y. Elkana, eds., 177–212. Dordrecht, Holland: D. Reidel Publishing Co.
    1989   Disabling practitioners: Hazards of learning to be a doctor in American medical education. *American Journal of Orthopsychiatry* 59:303–309.
Gordon, D.
    1988   Tenacious assumptions in Western medicine. In *Biomedicine examined*, M. Lock and D. Gordon, eds. Dordrecht, Holland: Kluwer.
Gottfried, R.
    1983   *The black death.* New York: Free Press.
Guarnaccia, P., and P. Farias
    1988   The social meanings of nervios: A case study of a Central American woman. *Social Science and Medicine* 26:1223–1231.
Guck, T., F. Skultely, P. Meilman, and E. Dowd
    1986   Prediction of long term outcome of multidisciplinary pain treatment. *Archives of Physical Medicine and Rehabilitation* 67:293–296.
Hallowell, A. I.
    1955   *Culture and experience.* New York: Schocken Books.
Hammonds, W., S. Brena, and I. Unikel
    1978   Compensation for work-related injuries and rehabilitation of patients with chronic pain. *Southern Medical Journal* 71:664–666.
Henryk-Gutt, R., and W. Rees
    1973   Psychological aspects of migraine. *Journal of Psychosomatic Research* 17: 141–153.
Herman, E., and S. Baptiste
    1981   Pain control: Mastery through group experience. *Pain* 10:79–86.
Hilbert, R.
    1984   The acultural dimensions of chronic pain: Flawed reality construction and the problem of meaning. *Social Problems* 31 (4): 365–378.
Hirschfield, A., and R. Behan
    1963   The accident process. I. Etiologic considerations of industrial injuries. *Journal of the American Medical Association* 186:193–199.
Hudgens, A.
    1979   Family-oriented treatment of chronic pain. *Journal of Marital and Family Therapy* 5:67–78.

Hughes, M., and K. Zimin
   1978   Children with psychogenic abdominal pain and their families. *Clinical
             Pediatrics* 17:569–573.
Jackson, J.
   n.d.   Report of fieldwork in chronic pain treatment settings. Manuscript.
James, W.
   1981   The consciousness of self. In *The principles of psychology*, 279–379. Cam-
   [1890]   bridge, Mass.: Harvard University Press.
Katon, W., A. Kleinman, and G. Rosen
   1982   Depression and somatization: A review. *American Journal of Medicine*
             72:127–134, 241–247.
Kaufman, S.
   1988   Toward a phenomenology of boundaries in medicine: Chronic ill-
             ness experience in the case of stroke. *Medical Anthropology Quarterly* 4:338–
             354.
Kerns, R., and D. Turk
   1984   Depression and chronic pain: The mediating role of the spouse. *Journal of
             Marriage and the Family* 46:845–852.
Kirmayer, L.
   1984   Culture, affect, and somatization. *Transcultural Psychiatric Research Review*
             21:159–188, 237–262.
   1988   Mind and body as metaphors: Hidden values in biomedicine. In *Biomedi-
             cine examined*, M. Lock and D. Gordon, eds., 57–93. Dordrecht, Holland:
             Kluwer.
Kleinman, A.
   1982   Neurasthenia and depression: A study of somatization and culture in
             China. *Culture, Medicine and Psychiatry* 6:117–191.
   1986   *Social origins of distress and disease.* New Haven, Conn.: Yale University
             Press.
   1988a   *The illness narratives: Suffering, healing and the human condition.* New York:
             Basic Books.
   1988b   *Rethinking psychiatry: From cultural category to personal experience.* New York:
             Free Press.
Kotarba, J.
   1983   *Chronic pain: Its social dimensions.* Beverly Hills, Calif.: Sage Publications.
Leavitt, F., D. Garron, W. Whisler, and M. Sheinkop
   1978   Affective and sensory dimensions of back pain. *Pain* 4:273–281.
Leff, J.
   1981   *Psychiatry around the globe.* New York: Marcel Dekker.
Leibman, R., P. Honig, and H. Berger
   1976   An integrated treatment program for psychogenic pain. *Family Process*
             15:397–406.
Levi, P.
   1961   *Survival in Auschwitz.* New York: MacMillan Publishing Co.
Lipowski, Z.
   1969   Psychosocial aspects of disease. *Annals of Internal Medicine* 71:1197–1206.

Lipton, J., and J. Marbach
    1984   Ethnicity and the pain experience. *Social Science and Medicine* 19:1279–1298.
Maruta, T., and D. Osborne
    1978   Sexual activity in chronic pain patients. *Psychosomatics* 20:241–248.
McBride, E.
    1965   Disability evaluation: The portage ticket to rehabilitation. *Archives of Physical Medicine* 46(suppl.): 115–120.
McHugh, S., and T. M. Vallis, eds.
    1986   *Illness behavior: A multidisciplinary model.* New York: Plenum Press.
McQueen, D., and J. Siegrist
    1982   Social factors in the etiology of chronic disease. *Social Science and Medicine* 16:353–367.
Mechanic, D.
    1972   Social psychological factors affecting the presentation of bodily complaints. *New England Journal of Medicine* 286:1132–1139.
Meissner, W.
    1974   Family process and psychosomatic disease. *International Journal of Psychiatric Medicine* 5:411–430.
Melzack, R.
    1973   *The puzzle of pain.* New York: Basic Books.
    1989   Phantom limbs, the self and the brain. *Canadian Psychology* 30:1–16.
Melzack, R., and W. Torgerson
    1971   On the language of pain. *Anesthesiology* 34:50–59.
Menges, L.
    1981   Psychological aspects of chronic pain. In *Persistent pain: Modern methods of treatment* (vol. 3), 5. Lipton and J. Miles, eds., 87–98. New York: Grune and Stratton.
Merskey, H.
    1987   Pain, personality and psychosomatic complaints. In *Handbook of Chronic Pain Management*, G. Burrows, D. Elton, and G. Stanley, eds., 137–146. Amsterdam: Elsevier Scientific Press.
Merskey, H., and F. Spear
    1967   *Pain: Psychological and psychiatric aspects.* London: Balliere, Tindall, and Cassel.
Migliore, S.
    1989   Punctuality, pain and time-orientation among Sicilian-Canadians. *Social Science and Medicine* 28(8): 851–860.
Miller, J.
    1976   Preliminary report on disability insurance. Public hearings before the subcommittee on Social Security of the Committee of Ways and Means, House of Representatives, 94th Congress, 2d Session, May–June 1976. Washington, D.C.: U.S. Government Printing Office.
Minuchin, S., B. Rosman, and L. Baker
    1978   The relationship of chronic pain to depression, marital adjustment, and family dynamics. *Pain* 5:285–292.

Morgan, L.
1987   Dependency theory in the political economy of health: An anthropo-
         logical critique. *Medical Anthropology Quarterly* 1:131–154.
Murphy, R.
1987   *The body silent.* New York: Henry Holt.
Ngor, H.
1987   *A Cambodian odyssey.* New York: MacMillan.
Oakeshott, M.
1985   *Experience and its modes.* Cambridge: Cambridge University Press.
[1933]
Obeyesekere, G.
1981   *Medusa's hair.* Chicago: University of Chicago Press.
Ohnuki-Tierney, E.
1981   *Illness and healing among the Sakhalin Ainu.* Cambridge: Cambridge Uni-
         versity Press.
Osterweis, M., A. Kleinman, and D. Mechanic, eds.
1987   *Pain and disability: Clinical, behavioral, and public policy perspectives.* Washing-
         ton, D.C.: National Academy Press.
Ots, T.
1990   The angry liver, the anxious heart, and the melancholy spleen: The
         phenomenology of perceptions in Chinese culture. *Culture, Medicine and
         Psychiatry* 4:21–58.
Pelz, M., and H. Merskey
1982   A description of the psychological effects of chronic painful lesions. *Pain*
         14:293–301.
Pilowsky, I.
1984   Pain and illness behavior: Assessment and management. In *Textbook of
         pain*, P. D. Walol and R. Melzack, eds. New York: Churchill Livingstone.
Pilowsky, I., and N. D. Spence
1976   Illness behavior syndromes associated with intractable pain. *Pain* 2:61–
         71.
Rosomoff, H., C. Green, M. Silbert, and R. Steele
1981   Pain and low back rehabilitation at the University of Miami School of
         Medicine. *NIDA Research Monograph* 36:92–111.
Salter, M., R. Brooke, H. Merskey, G. Fishter, and D. Kapusianyk
1983   Is the temporo-mandibular pain and dysfunction syndrome a disorder of
         the mind? *Pain* 17:151–166.
Scarry, E.
1985   *The body in pain.* New York: Oxford University Press.
Seres, J., J. Painter, and R. Newman
1981   Multidisciplinary treatment of chronic pain at the Northwest Pain Cen-
         ter. *NIDA Research Monograph* 36:41–65.
Shanfield, S., E. Heiman, D. Cope, and J. Jones
1979   Pain and the marital relationship: Psychiatric distress. *Pain* 7:343–351.
Sontag, S.
1989   *AIDS and its metaphors.* New York: Farrar, Strauss & Giroux.

Sternbach, R.
1968   *Pain: A psychophysiological analysis*. New York: Academic Press.
1974   *Pain patients: Tracts and treatments*. New York: Academic Press.
Stewart, D., and T. Sullivan
1982   Illness behavior and the sick in chronic disease. *Social Science and Medicine* 16:1397–1404.
Stone, D.
1984   *The disabled state*. Philadelphia: Temple University Press.
Susser, I., ed.
1988   Health and industry. Special issue of *Medical Anthropology Quarterly* 2(3).
Swanson, D.
1984   Chronic pain as a third pathological emotion. *American Journal of Psychiatry* 141:210–214.
Szasz, T.
1959   Language and pain. In *American handbook of psychiatry*, vol. 1, S. Arieti, ed. New York: Basic Books.
Tambiah, S.
1985   *Culture, thought, and social action*. Cambridge, Mass.: Harvard University Press.
Taylor, C.
1985   *Philosophical papers I: Human agency and language*. Cambridge: Cambridge University Press.
1989   *Sources of the self*. Cambridge, Mass.: Harvard University Press.
Turk, D., and H. Flor
1987   Pain > pain behavior: The utility and limitations of the pain behavior construct. *Pain* 31:277–295.
Turk, D., H. Flor, and T. Rudy
1987   Pain and families. I. Etiology, maintenance, and psychosocial impact. *Pain* 30:3–27.
Turkat, I., A. Kuczmierczyk, and H. Adams
1984   An investigation of the etiology of chronic headache: The role of headache models. *British Journal of Psychiatry* 145:665–666.
Turner, R. J., and S. Noh
1988   Physical disability and depression. *Journal of Health and Social Behavior* 29:23–37.
Turner, V.
1974   *Dramas, fields and metaphors: Symbolic action in human society*. Ithaca, N.Y.: Cornell University Press.
Venters, M.
1981   Familial coping with chronic and severe childhood illness: The case of cystic fibrosis. *Social Science and Medicine* 15A:289–297.
Violon, A.
1985   Family etiology of chronic pain. *International Journal of Family Therapy* 7:235–246.
Violon, A., and E. Giurgea
1984   Familial models for chronic pain. *Pain* 18:199–203.

Vrancken, M. A. E.
  1989   Schools of thought on pain. *Social Science and Medicine* 29(3): 435–444.
Warner, R.
  1985   *Recovery from schizophrenia: Psychiatry and political economy.* London: Rout-
            ledge & Kegan Paul.
Weighill, V.
  1983   Compensation neurosis: A review of the literature. *Journal of Psychosomatic
            Research* 27:97–104.
Weinstein, M.
  1968   The illness process: Psychosocial hazards of disability programs. *Journal
            of the American Medical Association* 204:209–213.
White, G.
  1982   The role of cultural explanations in "somatization" and "psychologiza-
            tion." *Social Science and Medicine* 16:1519–1530.
Work Disability in the United States
  1980   A Chartbook, U.S. Department of Health and Human Services, Social
            Security Administration Office of Research and Statistics. Washington,
            D.C.: U.S. Government Printing Office; Library of Congress Catalog
            Card No. 80-600183.
Yelin, E., et al.
  1980   Toward an epidemiology of work disability. *Milbank Memorial Fund
            Quarterly* 58(3): 386–414.
Zborowski, M.
  1952   Cultural components in response to pain. *Journal of Social Issues* 8(4): 16–
            31.
  1969   *People in pain.* San Francisco: Jossey-Bass.
Zola, I.
  1982   *Missing pieces: A chronicle of living with a disability.* Philadelphia: Temple
            University Press.

CHAPTER TWO

A Body in Pain—The Making of
a World of Chronic Pain[1]

Byron J. Good

"Doctor, is it possible that an experience in childhood can cause pain like his?" I was greeted by a sixty-four-year-old man bringing his twenty-eight-year-old son for an interview. The older man was tall and fairly thin, with a sagging face that showed sadness and concern. The younger man looked even less than his twenty-eight years. He walked rather stiffly, his face frozen and expressionless, perhaps, I thought, the result of medications. I deflected the question about childhood experience and asked them to join me and sit down, outlined our study of the experience of pain, explained that I was an anthropology professor, not a physician and not a therapist, and invited the younger man, whom I'll call Brian, to participate in the study.[2] He agreed readily, and with his permission, I invited his father to remain for the interview.

What followed was a remarkable story of a life of pain—a pain with an incredible origin myth, a pain that radically shaped the life world of a young man, a pain for which he struggled to find meaning and a language for expression. I spoke with Brian and his father only one time, for nearly four hours. The transcribed text of that interview serves as the basis for the following analysis. Interviews with other persons who participated in the pain studies described in this book also provide grounds for my reflections.

Elaine Scarry, in a brilliant discussion of the nature of pain and torture, argues that acute pain resists language (Scarry 1985). It is expressed in cries and shrieks, in a presymbolic language, resisting entry into the world of meaning. It "shatters" language, she says (p. 5); indeed, "intense pain is world-destroying" (p. 29). But such destruction is countered by a human response to find meaning, "to reverse the de-objectifying work of pain by forcing *pain itself* into avenues of objectification" (p. 6). "To witness the moment when pain causes a reversion to the pre-language of cries and groans is to witness the destruction of language; but conversely, to be present when a person moves up out of that pre-language and projects the facts of sentience into speech is almost to have been permitted to be present at the birth of language itself" (p. 6).

There are moments when interviewing a person in pain is indeed like witnessing the birth of language, as that person struggles to put into words an experience that resists language, a primal experience of the body that is at once ultimately real and ultimately indescribable, a force that so shapes the world that sufferers often describe themselves as inhabiting a world that others can never know. But language is not only inadequate when the intensity of pain can be expressed only in cries and the contorted body; it is perhaps more typically inadequate as a sufferer seeks a name for his pain, an individual name that accurately represents that pain, describes it with such clarity that its origins and contours are expressed, a representation possessing enough power that the pain can be controlled.

In a classic account of the Dinka, a Nilotic people of southern Sudan, Godfrey Lienhardt (1961) describes the response to members of the culture who are suddenly possessed. Ajak, a young man with his own incredible origin myth—he was born without testicles and was about to be put into the river by his father; instead, the infant's father was prevailed upon by his mother to offer a white sheep in sacrifice to divinity, whereupon first one, then the other testicle appeared—was suddenly possessed by a power. He ran wildly for twenty minutes and finally collapsed, sprawling on the ground. Lienhardt describes the response (p. 59):

> Then a minor master of the fishing-spear came and, addressing what he said to the thrashing form of Ajak, asked whatever it was which troubled him to tell its name and say what it wanted. In his address he tried to elicit answers from several potential sources of possession, saying, "You, Power" (*yin jok*), "You, divinity" (*yin yath*), and "You, ghost" (*yin atiep*). No reply, however, came from Ajak, who continued to moan and roll about. The master of the fishing-spear then began to take to task the Power which troubled Ajak, as follows: "You, Power (*jok*), why do you seize a man who is far away from his home? Why do you not seize him there at home where the cattle are? What can he do about it here?" . . .
>
> Ajak mumbled unintelligibly; the spectators were clearly expecting something to speak through his mouth, and to tell us its name and business. They explained that in due course it would leave him (*pal*). When I asked what "it" was, I was told variously that it would be his (clan) divinity (*yath*), or the ghost of his father, or the free-divinity Deng, or "just a Power" (*jok epath*). Since it would not announce itself, how could one know?

The naming of the source of suffering, particularly for those in chronic pain, often resembles this mysterious scenario. What is your name? Why are you troubling this person? the physicians seem to be asking. The response is often unintelligible. "It" refuses to speak. And if it will not announce itself, how can one know? The young man to which this essay bears witness was possessed of such an entity. The pain was unspeakable. It shaped a world. And it has resisted symbolization, refused to answer to a name, though many names have been proposed. It thus remains both untamed and ultimately unshared, for as Scarry says, "pain comes unsharably into our midst as at once that which cannot be denied and that which cannot be confirmed" (p. 4).

The story of Brian will be told in three parts: the origin myth and history of pain (the narrative); the shaping of a world of pain (the phenomenology); and the struggle for a name (the symbolization).

THE ORIGIN MYTH: NARRATING A LIFE IN PAIN

Brian was invited to participate in our study because he was a member of a health maintenance organization's support group for persons suffering chronic illness. After asking a few brief questions about his personal and family background, I asked him to tell me about his problem, to tell me the story about when it began and how he had tried to treat it. The narrative that evolved represented an effort to give shape to the pain, to name its origins in time and space, to construct a biography that made sense of a life of suffering (cf. this definition of illness narrative with that in Kleinman 1988).

He had a clear name for his pain—"I describe it as TMJ" ("temporomandibular joint disorder")—and a moment of diagnosis—"fall of 1984. I'd say November approximately." His TMJ was first diagnosed by a general physician treating him for difficulty breathing and pain in his ear, who "asked me to do some things with my jaw, move it up and down a few times. At that time, you could hear, hear a knocking and a clicking. I'd open up my jaw and at a certain point there'd be a snap, and then close again. So, that's when he, he made the initial diagnosis."[3]

But the description of his pain and its history quickly eluded ordered characterization, spilling out into his life.

> It seems like a long story now. When I became aware of it, it seemed like it might have had a very long history because I always seemed to have these things happening to me. I'd encounter dizzy spells and not know why I'd had them. . . . I was depressed and would just always be seeing counselors, would always be in a therapist's office for one reason or another. Then, [I had] the headaches, the dizzy sensations, sometimes had nausea that accompanies it. . . . It erupts in different places in your body. It comes in my head, then I have pains in my chest, I don't know what that's all about . . . it might be an anxiety attack, maybe get heart palpitations. And, ah, sensations of weakness, I, I, usually it affects my left side, the left side of my body is weaker than the other, than the right.

Words began to fail.

So really, ah, I'm a mess . . . seeing if I remember . . . I just couldn't seem to
move anywhere, I couldn't get myself to function very well. The, ah, I remember working . . . and standing for a long period of time and I just had a, an
attack of dizziness and [I didn't know] what, you know, what it was all about.
And it, it, for anybody that has TMJ, when it starts radiating and going into
your joints and going, traveling around inside your body, it's like a heat   it's a
burning type of a heat, and, ah, wrenching, and you feel it traveling along and
then it   you get things in your chest and you don't know what that's about,
and   you feel, ah, dizzy, you need, ah, shallow breathing type of thing   then I
thought I'd, well, dizziness I bet, there's been a history, there's been diabetes in
the family, maybe that's what I'm suffering from. I have low blood sugar. . . . I
can see why there might be some   relationship over that period of time to the,
eventually being diagnosed as having TMJ because ah, I did have Bruxism. I
was a   grinder. I grind my teeth at night, during my sleep. I would do it
during the day. It would just be, ah, a reflex I   if there was some   stress I
didn't know how to deal with, I'd internalize it for some reason and, ah, not
know that the way I was expressing it was by clenching my mouth. And then,
the, these teeth are very   crowded together. I'd rub the lower against the upper and just keep doing it over and over again   it seemed to   be a way of
handling anger or stress or something like that.[4]

But when did it all begin? "It might have . . . begun in adolescence, although
it became more pronounced as, uh, as I got older, the, the extreme nature of
it became more evident. . . " But did you seek treatment for it in high school?
"I hadn't even thought of it or interpreted it as a physical problem." As
psychological? "Even before I entered high school I think I was seeing therapists, and even when I was a child I was seeing therapists." So you have a
long history with psychological counselors? "A very long history." Since the
time your father mentioned, since you were two? "Yeah."

So the origins have space and time. The truly acute pains, it appears in
retrospect, originate in the body, in the jaw. They began in adolescence,
though it is hard to determine which childhood pains may have been a manifestation of TMJ. And before that, the origins are ultimately from the age of
two.

There are no secrets here, no mysteries to find voice for the first time. A
generation of therapists have heard the story. But it remains primeval,
mysterious.

At about that time, Mother had become gravely ill and she wasn't able to take
care of me, and Father didn't feel in a place where he could do . . . a good job of
it either. He didn't want to have relatives come on the scene and take care of
me. So, there was . . . an orphanage of some sort.   So I spent a period of three
months when I was two years of age and   it might have just come in right at
that time   that stripped me of any parental attachment. And ah, it was very

traumatic. I have no conscious memory of it, but something that damaged my feelings in the process . . . the only reason why I would have an inkling that that's where it all stems from is because I'd have these unexplained panicky feelings sometimes that I have to try something new, I have to be unafraid of authority, and I can't be and I feel intimidated. And so my, my initial in- clination was to withdraw, to, to develop a defense against all these perceived problems what I considered a threat.

And so a story took shape. The mother of this small child had hepatitis and was hospitalized. His father chose to leave him not in the care of family members but in the care of an orphanage. (Said his father: "With me it was just thick-headed pride. I didn't want my family in on the deal. But now I wish I had.") The infant emerged three months later completely changed, a "zombie." Brian was considered to be of above average intelligence in his childhood, but he was extremely sensitive and suffered spells of anxiety, of panic. "There's no legitimate reason to be very frightened, and yet suddenly I have an unexplained attack of anxiety," he says. He remembers the years between age nine and eleven as the only period relatively free of pain, as years "that I enjoyed life a little more." He has seen therapists for much of his life, beginning when he was two years old.

During adolescence Brian began to have pain—increasingly intense pain, "chronic headaches, radiating pains in and around my head, in the ear ca- nal, and my throat." He had spasms in his mouth and felt he was being choked. His depression and spells of anxiety continued; he would get an- xious, dizzy, feel the terror of losing control. And then, "over a long period of time the depression sets in, the chronic malaise and fatigue." He has been treated with antidepressant and antianxiety medications and was taking both at the time of the interview. The mysterious events within the walls of the orphanage, hidden from view and prior to symbolized memory, are in- scribed in his personal history as well as his body, evoking terror unmitigated by medication or psychotherapy.

Overlapping this narrative of a life in pain, a second narrative unfolds. In 1984, experiencing congestion and pain in his ears, Brian went to his general practitioner, thinking he had an ear infection. This physician heard a click- ing of his jaw and suggested this might account for his ear pain. Brian was referred to an ear, nose, and throat specialist, who treated his congestion but also "heard this pronounced clicking and popping sound" and "suggested that I had TMJ." Finally, a few months later, an ENT specialist at a tertiary care clinic examined him, explained the role of a deviated septum in ob- structing his breathing passages, and "while discussing that anatomy, he was also telling me about my jaw, the clicking that's going on inside there is a TMJ type of disorder. It's a malfunction of the jaw." Thus began a reinter- pretation of his pain. "I was still a little bit skeptical about the whole thing." But when the third consecutive physician mentioned the problem, "I said, well now, there's just no way of ducking it anymore." As a consequence, "I began to think that this is something that may have a physical basis in my jaw that I'd better start looking into   actually see where it leads me, and the whole idea was   one of hope, I guess, because now I had pinpointed something and defined it in a way. I can say that it's in my head, but it's not *all* in my head."

Brian was referred by one of his ENT specialists to a dentist specializing in "restorative dentistry." The dentist diagnosed his pain as arising from an occlusion problem—"I just wasn't biting properly." He ground several teeth to adjust the bite, then made a hard acrylic splint or occlusal device which fit snugly around the teeth and "relieved the stress in and around the ears." Unfortunately, forced to carry the devices along to work to wear part-time during the day, Brian lost the first device, then misplaced a second. Each time the dentist went through a long process of taking impressions, building a model, fitting and refitting the device, shaping, molding, and grinding it, at a cost to Brian of $350 per splint. When he lost or misplaced the device, Brian would feel humiliated and increasingly anxious, then fly into a rage. The more angry he became, the more the instances would repeat. Nonetheless, Brian continued in treatment with this dentist for nearly a year. He experienced some relief and began to feel hopeful, before doubts set in again.

> I think during the summer of that year, I began to think that I had an understanding of what was causing . . . why I was feeling terrible. . . . I actually had some clear image. . . . I knew what it was. I wasn't groping in the dark. It wasn't ambiguous anymore. It wasn't a whole lot of things.

And did that continue?

> Yeah, I guess that general outlook, that sense of hopefulness, continued for a period of time, and then I guess by the time I'd had my third appliance made, I began to, doubts set in again. I'd get worried. I still have headaches and what can they do about that? And before I could see a physical therapist, I needed a referral from a doctor, so he was the one who made the referral.

The most recent major treatment that Brian has undergone has been at the hands of a private physical therapist who does deep tissue massage. Rather than just his jaw, his entire body has been the object of treatment. "It seemed like every part of my body had some relationship to what was happening. . . . It was my chest. It was my back. It was my legs. . . . Then my whole notion of what was going on began to change again: maybe it isn't as simple as I had initially thought." The therapist used extremely painful techniques aimed at "releasing" areas of stress in tissues that were bound up, tight, and jammed. The first several months of treatment led to "activation" and "upset" of his viscera, with his attacks of heartburn becoming especially intense. Over the next several months, treatments became more subtle, and

Brian experienced some relaxation. Finally, treatments were reduced from several each week, to weekly, to once every several weeks, and the treatments were concluded a month before the interview. Although some of the tension has been reduced and the physical therapist felt her work was complete, Brian continues to have intense pain in his head, neck, back, and legs. He continues to seek care.

The most recent consultation was three days before our interview. At the suggestion of his internist, who treats his gastrointestinal problems, Brian set up an appointment with and was examined by an oral surgeon in one of the local teaching hospitals. "Panoramic X-rays" were taken, but Brian reported that, according to the surgeon, they didn't "reveal any real abnormal things that require surgery." The surgeon recommended that he go back to wearing his splint regularly to protect against his clenching his jaws and grinding his teeth. He placed a great deal of emphasis on stress alleviation and relaxation and recommended meditation and exercise. "And how did this strike you?" I asked.

> Well, it sort of was an answer I may have been able to give myself actually. I didn't need to see a specialist for that. . . . It sort of goes back to a little more holistic approach. It's more involved; it's back to an ambiguity again. And then it goes back into my conflict about my body. Is it my body? Is it my thinking process that activates physical stresses? Or am I, or is it the other way around? It's all that uncertainty that. . . .

"No magic bullet," I said.

> Yeah, no magic bullet. Every time I look for one, I seem to encounter just another maze or morass of things.

And so now? What lies ahead in this narrative? "Right at this stage, I'm grappling with a lot of despair," Brian says quietly.

> I still have pain on occasion and now I'm also questioning again. Is it really TMJ, or am I, or is it something that, ah, is it an emotional disturbance that's more the issue that I have to deal with? And once I get into a state of confusion like that, uncertainty and, ah, I guess, this hopelessness, the sort of generalized feeling of, ah, empty type of feeling, what am I going to do now?

THE WORLD UNMADE: THE PHENOMENOLOGY

Elaine Scarry describes pain as "shattering" language, as "world-destroying." In the horror of the torture chambers that she analyzes, language is literally shattered, reduced to cries and shrieks. For many pain patients, language is anything *but* shattered in this literal sense. Brian was wonderfully and frighteningly articulate, though language at times seemed inadequate to express the sentient quality of his suffering. As he sat stiffly and quietly, he described an amazing and rich inner world. At the same time, as we will explore in this section, his pain shapes his world to itself, resisting objectification and threatening the objective structure of the everyday world in which Brian participates.

BG: How would you describe what's going on inside your body?

BRIAN: Sometimes, if I had to visualize it, it would seem as though there, there, there's a, ah, ama, a demon, a monster, something very horro, horrible lurking around banging the insides of my body, ripping it apart. And ah, I'm containing it, or I'm trying to contain it, so that no one else can see it, so that no one else can be disturbed by it. Because it's scaring the daylights out of me, and I'd assume that   gee, if anybody had to, had to look at this, that ah, they'd avoid me like the plague. So I redouble my efforts to   say . . . I'm gonna be perfectly contained about this whole thing. And maybe the less I do, the less I make myself known, and the less I, I ah, I venture out or, or display any, any initiative, then I won't let the, this junk out. It seems like there's something very, very terrible happening. I have no control over it, it's ah   I really don't have any control over it, although I like to believe I do. At least to the extent that nobody else is going to   because if they find out, then   they won't believe me, but on the one hand, if you start talking about it, or they'll ah, they'll have their own   their own answers and ahm, solutions that don't jive with your own. So, I guess that's   a fairly accurate way of describing it   the pain gets really terrible   there's no way to   really convey it or talk to about it, or talk about it with anyone. Sometimes, I just go into head trips and rationalization in my mind trying to explain it away, trying to say that it's all just imaginary, it's a figment, it really doesn't exist. And that's a, becomes a mechanism for handling it. If I convince myself in an intellectual way that it's not there, or it's not really important enough or, ah, I'm making too much out of this, ah   then it, you know, I won't fall apart. I won't, ah, be so totally dysfunctioning that . . . I won't be able to do anything again.

Through his rich description, Brian provides us access to a world of pain. It is a shocking world of monsters ripping apart his body, a private world he fears to share with others, a world they could not possibly understand, and yet a world absolute and inescapable for him, which he wants desperately to construe as imaginary but cannot. At the same time, through great determination, Brian has continued to go to work at an insurance company every day. He lives with his family, attends meetings of the support group, visits physicians and therapists, attends school at night, and is a painter. What do we mean by invoking the term *world* in this context? Does it make sense to speak of the world of the chronic pain sufferer? In what way is the world of the pain sufferer a special, private, even unsharable world? What are the characteristics of that world? In what way can chronic pain be said to "unmake" the world for the sufferer?

The term *world* as used here is linked to a long history of phenomenologically oriented philosophers and social scientists—from Edmund Husserl, Maurice Merleau-Ponty, and Sartre to Nelson Goodman, and from William James to Alfred Schutz and various contemporary sociologists and anthropologists. For Husserl, the "life world," the *Lebenswelt*, is the world of our common, immediate, lived experiences. This world is often contrasted with the objective world of the sciences, and many assume that the latter represents reality in the strict sense of the word. Husserl and like-minded social scientists have argued that rather than the life world presupposing this scientific world, the obverse is true. Science is grounded in the life world. It assumes a particular perspective, a particular attitude to be taken toward reality, and it constitutes a distinctive scientific world, but it presupposes dimensions of experience and its interpretation common to the life world. The scientific world is only one of several worlds or "subuniverses" in which we live, worlds that include those of religious experience, of dreams and fantasies, of music and art, and of the "common-sense" reality that is paramount in much of our lives. Furthermore, though the life world can be investigated in relation to individual experience, it is an intersubjective world, a social and cultural world, a world that resists our desire to shape it at our own whims, a world of social facts and realities that we cannot wish away.

How can we approach an understanding of the world of chronic pain? We return to Husserl's description of method:

> I begin . . . by questioning that which has in me, under the heading "world," the character of the conscious, the experienced, and the intended, and which is accepted by me as being; I ask what it looks like in its being accepted thus; I ask how I become conscious of it, how I may describe it . . . ; how what is subjective in this way manifests itself in different modes, what it looks like in itself, . . . how it is to be described, what kind of achievement it is that brings about in me a world of this typical existential character. (Husserl, quoted in Brand 1967:209)

That is, we explore the organization of sentience, of experience, as well as the objects of experience, the contours of the world as experienced and responded to, as well as the organization and shaping of experience. Here we will examine Brian's description of his suffering and of the world in which he lives, contrasting it with the world of everyday reality as described by Alfred Schutz, and return to Scarry's observation that pain has the singular power to destroy worlds.

In Brian's description, bodily experience assumes enormous proportions. He begins by describing the pain arising from the jaw joint, but it quickly eludes narrow characterization, as he describes the anxiety engendered and his attacks of panic. This merges again into his description of pain.

> It goes into the head . . . inside my mouth would be hot because the spasming was going into my mouth and down where I would be swallowing and I wanted

something to relax it. . . . The, the maxillary muscles in the roof of my mouth
would get all tightened up, and so I had to drink something warm to relax it.
And it goes down here, and people would describe it as being choked or having
this lump of this sensation of being restricted all the way through here. [He
gestured to his throat and chest.] And it starts going down. And then as your
anxiety builds, you don't know what the heck is going on, and you start feeling
other things, and sensations of heartburn and ah, sometimes, I get dizzy
along with that. I start to breathe more rapidly. . . . The scariest part of it is that
I'm losing control, I, I'm suddenly finding that not be able to contain myself
anymore I don't know what's happening because it's so, so, so strange I
attributed, ah, weakness in my leg to that and having stress in one leg more
than the other it's always my left hand that seems to be have more pain in it
than in the, these, ah, muscle cramps that go down my, ah, left arm, and
sometimes a numb sensation in my hand. . . . Seems like at the worst moments,
all my symptoms are, ah, prevalent I have to do something. I've gotta get
things done. I'm, ah, I'm working and, ah, why do I have to, have to have the
allness of this type of, of affliction.

The pain at times builds up, and "streaks" about his body.

Usually it's like a pressure building up. It starts to move around and travel as
if it were a hot streak, lightning or something like that. . . . I'll feel twinges in
my shoulder, in the vertebrae that, that run down the neck and the spinal
column or it may, may go down to my arm, and then, ah, a whole separate
problem with the stomach disorders has been cropping up recently, but I'm
not sure what the exact nature of the relationship between that and TMJ is. It's
not supposed to be, but I've had irregularity . . . and a lot of stomach discomfort and cramping in that part of my body.

In Brian's world, the body has special primacy, as he eloquently describes. It absorbs the world into itself, floods out into the world and shapes
not only his experience but the experienced world. Brian struggles to continue to work, but it is just when "I've gotta get things done" that the "allness of this type of affliction" threatens to overwhelm him. As a consequence,
he said, "I'm at a stage where I could very well quit work. . . . Sometimes I
think I'm working through a nervous breakdown. . . . As long as I fool people, they don't know what's going on . . . I won't be carted away someplace.
But it's a tremendous effort. Sometimes I question if I can keep it up." Thus,
Brian is unable to simply live through his body in the "world of everyday
life," in the "world of working" (Schutz 1971:208–229), directing his attention to practical ends, whether set by himself or those who have turned the
workplace into what he calls a kind of "chain gang." His body comes to
dominate consciousness, threatening to unmake the everyday world, and it is
only through "tremendous effort" that he can attend to what is for most of us
our paramount world.

Schutz (1971:216) argues that in the everyday world, the self is experienced as the "author" of its activities, as the "originator" of our ongoing actions, and thus as an "undivided total self." We act in the world *through* our bodies; our bodies are the subject of our actions, that through which we experience, comprehend, and act upon the world. In contrast, Brian described his body as having become an object, distinct from the experiencing and acting self. He articulated several dimensions of this. The pain has agency. It is a demon, a monster, lurking around, banging the insides of his body. Pain is an "it" that "erupts in various places in your body," that streaks around the body, which Brian seldom feels able to control. Pain is also fundamentally aversive. It is, in Scarry's terms, "a pure physical experience of negation, an immediate sensory rendering of 'against,' of something being against one. . . . Even though it occurs within oneself, it is at once identified as 'not oneself,' 'not me,' as something so alien that it must right now be gotten rid of" (1985:52). At the same time, pain is a part of the subject, a dimension of the body, a part of the self. As a consequence, the body itself becomes aversive agent. "I think it's against me, that I have an enemy," Brian said of his body. "My own physical body isn't going to cooperate. It's just gonna always let me down."

> BG: Do you have a sense in some ways that you think more of your body as a kind of object? That is, that it somehow is not really you?
>
> BRIAN: Yeah. I've never even noticed those moments too when I think it's . . . I'm outside myself, this whole thing I've got to deal with is, ah, a decayed mass of tissue that's just not any good, and I, I'm almost looking at it that way again; as if my mind were separated from my self, I guess. I don't feel integrated. I don't feel like a whole person because I'm always grappling with some type of physical defect . . . and then I can get to see myself as defective. . . . I'm disabled, I'm dysfunctional, I'm whatever, whatever else you want to, label you want to pin on it. And then I get angry about that too, you know.

Thus, as locus of pain, the body takes on agency over and against the self. It becomes a "decayed mass of tissue" that is separated from the self, and the undivided total self becomes defective and loses integration.

One of the most fundamental assumptions of the everyday life is that we live in the same world as persons around us, that the world we experience and inhabit is shared by others (see Schutz 1971:218–222). For many persons with chronic illness, this assumption is called into doubt. Their world is experienced as different, as a realm that others cannot fully fathom. For the sufferer of pain, this sense is often particularly acute. Pain resists the objectification of standard medical testing; there are no pain meters, no biochemical assays for pain. It resists *localization*; most efforts to identify the site of the origin of chronic pain fail, despite all advances in imaging techniques, and nearly all surgical attempts to remove pain pathways are quickly undone by the body's efficient generation of new pathways. As Ronald Melzack wrote in 1973, the concept of a pain center in the brain is "pure fiction, unless virtually the whole brain is considered to be the pain centre" (quoted in Scarry 1985:55). At the same time, although it is experienced with absolute and often searing certainty, pain resists the objectification of language, the confirmation of social consensus. As quoted earlier in this chapter, Brian described feeling the need to be "perfectly contained," because "if they find out . . . they won't believe me" or "they'll have their own answers and solutions that don't jive with your own." He described this more directly later in the interview.

> BG: Do you ever have a sense that you live in a world that is different from that of other people? Perhaps a world that other people really can't understand?

> BRIAN: Ahm, yeah. That's the overall feeling that I have. People really can't understand the TMJ person at all. If they don't suffer with it, they don't understand it. And they're really skeptical. They don't believe in you. They think you're just a little bit different and strange. Ahm, sort of, ahm, a misfit; you're just not, or I guess, inscrutable. They can't understand it. They don't know what it is. Maybe this is just something you're making up.

Others believe this world to be "made up." Brian desperately wishes he could believe it to be so, that he could "explain it away . . . say that it's all just imaginary, it's a figment, it really doesn't exist." He cannot do so. On the contrary, pain is the central reality; it dominates experience and expression. It "monopolizes language, becomes its only subject: complaint . . . becomes the exclusive mode of speech" (Scarry 1985:54). Verbal objectification, the extension of the self into the world, and thus the self authored in the process, is dominated by pain. But since others doubt the word, they doubt the world and its author. "They think you're . . . different . . . strange . . . inscrutable." The usual suspension of doubt which allows us to accept one another's account of the world, what Schutz calls the "*epoche* of the natural attitude" (Schutz 1971:229), is withheld from the accounts of the pain sufferer. As a consequence, the self and the world of the pain sufferer are threatened with dissolution.

Our dialogue continued:

> BG: What's the nature of that world that they can't understand?

> BRIAN: I don't know, for me it's, ah, it's a constriction. It's being bound up, ah, just having a pained body and not being able to adequately explain it or interpret it. Knowing I can't, it's so overall, so pervasive, I can't really say, yes it's like a headache, but it's not like a headache either. You have to have it to really understand what it's like. You have to find out what it's like to come home and feel you don't know what time of the day it is. Even though you have a watch right in front of you, you don't know what time of the day it is. You have to lay

down just because, ah, you feel you're going to be crushed any minute because the pain is so bad, or that it, you don't know if there's gonna, if you're going to wake up in the morning if you go to sleep. You're just so fearful. There's a sensation you have, you have it's a total thing I've had these sensations, and the head is being clamped inside a vice, and something's jamming me on one side or the other and just a wheel is being cranked all the time, and so it goes on. It goes around my head and then, it's kind of strange when I come home at night and I lay down for fifteen minutes. I might drift off into sleep and I might not, but I'm sort of in an in-between state and, ah, everything seems sort of almost, if not I can, well the fantasies going around in my head. Usually, I've had a stressful day, and I lay down for fifteen minutes, but then I won't know whether half an hour has passed or a whole day, or, ah, three or four hours. Time becomes distorted.

Time seems distorted. Not only is social validation of the experience of the pain sufferer withheld, threatening the taken-for-granted quality of the life world, but the building blocks of the perceived world—time, space—begin to dissolve. Schutz (1971:214–218) argues that in everyday life our personal experience of time, of inner time (which Schutz calls *duree*), is synchronized with outer time, with time as socially organized and validated. The life world we share with others is experienced as having a common time structure. This is far more subtle than we often imagine, as becomes clear when persons discover they have life-threatening illness and begin to reassess time. Such persons often report experiencing time differently than those around them; time is short, not to be wasted, experienced with impatience. For Brian, inner and outer time seem out of sync. Even more terrifying, time itself seems to break down, to lose its ordering power. The interview continued:

BG: I was actually going to ask about that. Does time seem any different to you than it did before, or than it does for other people?

BRIAN: For me, yeah, time seems to be spreading out, almost like I can't say anything is happening now. I have no way of pigeonholing a specific span of time which I can get a few things done. Seems like I'm usually losing track of it. I can't keep up with it. Or it's all, everything's caving in on me at once; the past, the present are coming together all at one time. . . . episodes that repeat over and over again: you know, physical episodes of pain that seem to repeat. I can remember a time in the past when you've had it, and you can't even distinguish now from then. You really get a very warped and distorted view of what time is. So, that's sort of, a very disturbing aspect of it.

BG: Does time seem slower or faster? Or are there times, are there periods in your life when time seems to race or time seems to slow down?

BRIAN: Usually time seems to race when I'm racing; when I'm in the throes of some kind of activity I want to get done, time is racing by very fast. Or there's something that I'm not filling up with that time, the time is rushing by anyway.

I haven't done anything. I may have been bogged down because I have these pains to deal with, or I just don't feel up to it, and I regret that time has gone, and I haven't done anything with it. And it seems to have gone before I had, it seems to be moving too fast. I know rationally I have no way of controlling it. There might be some type of force of will which isn't really the, too good   tend to dictate. I'd like to be able to control it. I'd like to be able to get back some things I've missed out on or something.

Thus time caves in. Past and present lose their order. Pain slows personal time, while outer time speeds by and is lost. An act of will is required to order time, and time filled with pain is experienced as lost. Thus as articulate as Brian is about the world of pain, it cannot be sustained by language. It is a world threatened by dissolution. Space and time are overwhelmed by pain, and the private world not only loses its relation to the world in which others live, its very organizing dimensions begin to break down. Pain threatens to unmake the world.

In this context, Brian's repeated expressions of concern about "losing control" have special meaning. The word "control" appears thirteen times in the transcript at eight points in the interview. Twice he expresses concern about his ability to control pain or that monster banging about in his body. Once he describes himself as a "victim of life rather than someone who has some control over it." Once he describes his inability to control time, to regain what has been lost. And four times he discusses the terror that he may simply lose control:

I almost feel like I'm gonna reach a breaking point and then, ah, that'll be it. What if my super control and defense mechanisms aren't strong enough to keep me intact? And it does, and I do explode and I just go berserk and say, I can't tolerate it . . . I'll be outside and just lose control. I can't stand it anymore.

This theme expresses a profound fear of dissolution of the self and the experienced life world. The assumption that the world possesses stability is replaced by a sense of its arbitrariness, a feeling that will is required, that control is necessary to maintain the self and the world. Together with the attacks of panic and anxiety, the pain floods the consciousness, dominates inner time, and breaks down the ordered relationship between the conscious self and the world to which it relates. The pervasiveness of the body expands its boundaries, shuts out attention to the outer world, and threatens dissolution. Only by controlling and containing it—"So I redouble my efforts to . . . be perfectly contained about this whole thing"—can the self be maintained. But this effort to be contained is profoundly isolating, further threatening the self and its relation to the everyday world and intersubjectivity. Thus the world of chronic pain, the separate world inhabited by its sufferers, is at the same time a world unmade.

THE STRUGGLE FOR A NAME: THE SYMBOLIZATION

The Dinka treat members of their society who are possessed by calling forth the names of the Divinities—"You Power, you Divinity, you Ghost, why do you trouble this man"—waiting for one to answer to its name, to speak through the mouth of the sufferer, to announce its business and the sacrifice it requires. Lienhardt analyzes each of the Powers and Divinities as images grounded in discrete complexes of Dinka experience. For the Dinka, however, these Powers are themselves the grounds of experience, the source of power and the origins of certain forms of suffering. They are, says Lienhardt, central to the process of symbolization necessary for healing.

> Without these powers or images or an alternative to them there would be for the Dinka no differentiation between experience of the self and of the world which acts upon it. Suffering, for example, could be merely "lived" or endured. With the imagining of the grounds of suffering in a particular Power, the Dinka can grasp its nature intellectually in a way which satisfies them, and thus to some extent transcend and dominate it in this act of knowledge. With this knowledge, this separation of a subject and an object in experience, there arises for them also the possibility of creating a form of experience they desire, and of freeing themselves symbolically from what they must otherwise passively endure. (Lienhardt 1961:170)

The medical treatment for chronic pain is often like Dinka divination. A series of names are called out, and the diviner and sufferer alike wait for the power to announce itself. Medical treatment is aimed at constructing an image that names the origins of the pain in the sufferer's biography and its source in the sufferer's body. Unfortunately, as in the case of the young Dinka man described early in this chapter, the response is often unintelligible, the power refuses to reveal itself, or the physicians cannot agree upon the name of the power. However, chronic pain sufferers press on, constantly seeking a name for their suffering, an image that will name its source and allow it to be set off from the self, an image that will provide the symbolic structure for a remaking of the world.

For Brian, there were two names for his suffering, psyche and soma, stress or anxiety or depression and TMJ. One after another, these names have been called out, and sacrifices have been offered to each. The two are conflicting images, however, and to date neither has had the power to free him from his suffering.

For many years, Brian has been in therapy for psychological problems that began at age two. This narrative is a clear one. That mysterious period in the orphanage "stripped [him] of any parental attachment," left him with unexplained feelings of panic, fear of authority, a sense of being victimized, recurrent bouts of depression, and because of tension and teeth grinding, increasing and nearly unbearable pain. Unfortunately, this naming of his problem and the attendant therapies—both psychotherapy and medications—have not had the power to diminish the pain and suffering.

When he was twenty-four years old, a new name was proposed for his pain. Temporomandibular joint disorder (TMJ) or temporomandibular disorders (TMD) are conceived as disorders of the temporomandibular joints, which result in orofacial pain, limitations in range of motion accompanied by catching and locking of the jaw, and headaches, earaches, and cervical pain. It is often treated with appliances for bruxism, mandibular repositioning, and joint stabilization; anti-inflammatory medication and analgesics; and referral for dental and orthodontic treatment (see Von Korff et al. 1988*a* and 1988*b*). The suggestion that he had TMJ led Brian to reinterpret many of his problems, to revise the narrative of his illness.

> If I had earaches as a kid, or I had problems, then it could have, it could have been TMJ that far back. If I'd felt sick on occasion not knowing why, could that have been a TMJ problem? In my last year in high school, I remember I had vomited one morning and because I had, had woken up with just an incredible headache I was spinning around and very dizzy. It's only now in retrospective, I look back, could that have had something to do with TMJ?

At first, he was extremely hopeful. The pain had a clear origin in a specific site in the body, not simply in "stress" or "anxiety." It had a name that could explain many of his most debilitating and seemingly unconnected physical symptoms. There were TMJ specialists and recommended treatments. And the initial treatments seemed to provide some alleviation of the pain. However, as treatment progressed, the most severe symptoms remained. The range of treatments recommended by members of the TMJ support group grew. The answers became "more holistic," more "ambiguous," less clear. And Brian again began to despair.

At the time of the interview, Brian was caught between these two images of the source of his suffering. At the beginning of the interview, I asked about his depressions. He replied that only recently has he begun to think of them as resulting from his TMJ. "It seems to engender a lot of conflict for me, though, when I think of whichever came first. Is it, am I depressed and then I get my physical pain from that, or is it working reverse? And then I get, ah, very divided and conflicted over it, and then not sure what, what the right thing is to believe or where to go." When I asked when the TMJ began, he could not be clear: "I would think it was at least a decade or more." And what is the reason it began when it did?

> It may have been a physical thing that I've been doing with my teeth, the grinding and so forth it just, it may have also been a result of, ah, of being repressed or suppressing my emotions, not really, ah . . . sometimes I, I feel a victim of life rather than someone who has some control over and ah, more

manipulated I guess. . . . I'd never be vocal or out in the open with stress or anger. It would be internalized most of the time. Then I guess the way it manifested itself was, was teeth grinding and   sometimes, I'd physically clench other parts of my body, would stiffen up, I'd, my legs would become tight   that sort of thing.

But why the conflict? Why does the recognition of these two competing images for his disorder cause Brian such acute and explicit conflict? It is because, troubled as he is, Brian is psychologically sophisticated and painfully honest.

I'm always wondering if   my magical thinking will want to tell me I'd like to have a cure right now   that, that there is something out there, all I can do is   if it's a correction of, some surgeon can do that, then the problems are over, or I can take a, some medication and the problems are gone or, after I go through this massage treatment, the problems will evaporate. It doesn't.

BG: Pretty nice way to think.

BRIAN: Yeah, that's what I said. It's almost like a comforting way to think. You almost need to think like that in order to, to keep yourself stable somehow.

BG: In order to maintain some kind of hope that ultimately there is some way to deal with this.

BRIAN: Yeah. The flip side of the coin is that I could also appear, verge on despair at some points. And another thing is, cropping up in my mind is that it, hope that my worst fears aren't going to be   fulfilled in that I have to live with this forever.

The conflict Brian experiences is so great not only because of his honesty, because of his awareness of the seduction of magical thinking, but also because the consequences are so enormous. To name the origin of the pain is to seize power to alleviate it, and the intensity of the pain demands urgency. To name the origin of the pain is also a critical step in the remaking of the world. The conflict over narratives is a conflict over biographical construction. Is the pain an essential part of the self, or is it "merely" a part of the body? Can the pain be separated as object from the self as subject, thus differentiating the subject from the world that acts upon it, or must he "passively endure" the pain? The authoring of an integrated self depends on the answer to these questions. The conflict over interpretations is also the basis for developing a socially accepted and validated image of his problem. If TMJ is an accepted interpretation, the "reality" of his problem is more likely to be accepted. It is a medical problem, one with accepted objectivity, one accepted not only by specialists but by a community, members of the chronic-illness support group, who vouch for its objectivity and validity. It is the grounds for rebuilding a relationship to a consensual world, a means for reentering the everyday world. Ultimately the conflict is over the discovery of an effective name, an effective diagnosis that can serve as the basis for treatment and relief.

Unfortunately, at the time of the interview, the conflict remained unresolved. "It's back to an ambiguity again. And then it goes back into my conflict about my body. Is it my body? Is it my thinking process that activates physical stresses? Or am I, or is it the other way around? It's all that uncertainty." If you were to tell me where you currently stand, I asked near the end of the interview, how would you answer? "Right now, I haven't made a decision . . . but in my mind what I'd like to say is if I could tell myself that it was a physical thing, if I could just have a little less pain, I think I could handle some things if I just didn't have quite as much pain." And because of this hope, he keeps looking for answers. There is a surgeon recommended by a member of the support group. There is someone involved in a study at a pain center. The television program "20/20" describes the case of a woman who had a severe case of TMJ. She went through "a treatment program that lasted four days and was cured of the whole thing." "Pain-free," his father says. "Now she's pain-free," Brian says. "She still has the disorder, but she's come to not be as dysfunctional from it. You know, she's overcome a great amount of pain." The hope remains.

"It amazes me that amidst all these things," his father continues, "he can go do a piece of artwork and set it up, and what comes out is strictly individual and it's his artwork. Can't confuse it with any other." Brian is an artist. When language fails as a medium of self-extension, as "a vehicle through which the pain could be lifted out into the world and eliminated" (Scarry 1985:54), Brian turns to painting. For a while he did surrealist painting, and a lot of "bizarre sort of subconscious images" came out. Is there a way to at least embody your experience through art? I asked.

> Well, there are times when I, when a lot of things that are ineffable about what goes on internally, I can find expression in the art. A lot of bizarre things I can't verbalize come out in the images I get down on canvas. . . . If I have a shrieking person inside me, someone that's yelling and screaming and trying to get out, sometimes I don't do it concretely. You know, I don't do it verbally. I do it by   it comes out in the painting. . . .
>
> It's a way of resolving something. If I can't do it any other way, then I can do it through the painting. And it's better too. At least it's not bound up, and . . . I'm not holding on to it anymore.

> BG: Do you have a sense of release when you finish a painting?

> BRIAN: Sometimes, there's a bit of accomplishment. I feel good about it. . . . I hope it conveys a little bit of the feeling, a little bit of what the real depth of my experience is like, and somebody else can see it. And then sometimes, they do see it, and they ah . . . they seem to me to get very, ah, affected by it. But each time I do a painting, it's exposing a little piece of myself, so I have to know who it is that's going to understand it.

BG: Is that part of your unwillingness to sell your paintings or display them you think?

BRIAN: Yeah, I have to know . . . if it will be accepted. . . . If I reveal something about myself, something that can be, that is very vulnerable and, ah, is likely to be met with skepticism, people aren't going to understand it, or they're going to have a totally different impression, or they'll mock it in some way, so that's the kind of fear I have. And, ah, I can't show it to ordinary people that I come into contact with during the course of the day.

Thus, for Brian, painting provides a medium for objectification of that which cannot be expressed through language. He continues to seek medical treatment in order to find an image with the power to heal. This search is a form of symbolic action, an attempt to make real and objective his pain, and an attempt to author a self and a world in relation to a sensible image of pain. However, he is courageous enough to recognize the potential for mystification. And so he turns at times to the world of images, where the scream can be expressed without a sound, where the ineffable can find expression, where an extremely vulnerable self can venture into the world.

CONCLUSION

This chapter has been a reflection on a four-hour conversation with a single young man and his father. It cannot be said to represent the lives of the many who suffer either TMJ or chronic pain. It is meant, however, to bear witness to a single life and to an experience deeply resistant to language. Although more articulate than most, Brian described a world much akin to those described by other pain sufferers who participated in our studies. When pain is intense, the body dominates consciousness, "obliterating" its contents, as Scarry says. When pain is chronic, it extends into the world, shaping the world to itself. The world of pain becomes a special world, a world largely unshared and unsharable, inhabited by persons who have given up on revealing "that which cannot be denied and cannot be confirmed." Many continue actively in the everyday world of others, while they resist the threats of pain to "unmake" that world. The search for care is sometimes desperate, a seeming attempt to resist dissolution of the self and the world. Others seem unwilling to invest hope in the objectification of their pain in medical terms, having been too often disappointed by the names provided by medicine. For many, the contradictions of psyche and soma as images for the grounds of their suffering are near consciousness. Accepting psyche as the name for pain suggests to many that that which cannot be denied is unreal. Searching for soma as the name for chronic pain is often recognized to involve magical thinking, and even when a clear name, such as TMJ, is given, it remains untreatable. The demon within answers to neither name. Faced with this dilemma, many who suffer chronic pain persevere, suffering pain in relative solitude while courageously finding other media for self expression, whether in artistic creation or authoring professional lives or building families.

NOTES

1. The title of this chapter purposely reflects that of Elaine Scarry's book, *The Body in Pain: The Making and Unmaking of the World* (New York: Oxford University Press, 1985), which serves as the source for my reflections on the words of the young man whose life is described here.

2. Specific identifying characteristics of this young man have been altered to preserve confidentiality.

3. It is worth noting that Brian is in several ways *not* representative of persons we have interviewed who have been diagnosed as suffering TMJ. He has a long history of psychological problems, as he made clear in the interview, and he has suffered extreme and persistent pain through much of his body. Neither of these are characteristic of many persons who suffer jaw joint disorders (see, e.g., Von Korff et al. 1988*a*, 1988*b*). I chose to tell Brian's story in this book because of his chronic pain, rather than his diagnosis as a TMJ sufferer.

4. Triple periods (. . .) indicate words or sentences are omitted from the transcription. Extra space between words indicates a pause in Brian's speech.

REFERENCES CITED

Brand, Gerd
  1967   Intentionality, reduction, and intentional analysis in Husserl's later manuscripts. In *The philosophy of Edmund Husserl and its interpretation*, Joseph J. Cockelmans, ed., 197–217. Garden City, N.Y.: Doubleday & Co.
Kleinman, Arthur
  1988   *The illness narratives: Suffering, healing and the human condition.* New York: Basic Books.
Lienhardt, Godfrey
  1961   *Divinity and experience: The religion of the Dinka.* Oxford: Oxford University Press.
Scarry, Elaine
  1985   *The body in pain: The making and unmaking of the world.* New York: Oxford University Press.
Schutz, Alfred
  1971   On multiple realities. In *Collected papers I: The problem of social reality*, Maurice Natanson, ed., 207–259. The Hague: Martinus Nijhoff.
Von Korff, Michael, et al.
  1988*a*   Temporomandibular disorders: Variation in clinical practice. *Medical Care* 26:307–314.
  1988*b*   An epidemiological comparison of pain complaints. *Pain* 32:173–183.

CHAPTER THREE

Work as a Haven from Pain

Mary-Jo DelVecchio Good

The conventional model that dominates popular American discourse on the relationship between pain and work characterizes work as "stressful," producing or amplifying pain. It is not at all surprising that this linear model, so salient in popular American notions about health and illness, fosters investment in pain research based in related paradigms. Estimated medical costs of work "stress" now approach $100 billion per year, and vast resources have been expended on work disability payments for those who suffer from chronic pain (Karasek and Theorell 1990; Osterweis et al. 1987). Such expenditures and the national concern with "estimates" of the cost of work stress are brute documents of our culture's contemporary association of work with pain or ill health. Research with individuals who are afflicted with chronic pain, however, suggests that the historical association of work and *good* health, so central to American culture in the past, continues to have an everyday veracity and to play counterpoint to the late twentieth-century refrain of "work → stress → ill health."[1]

The meaning of work in the lives of active professionals who suffer from chronic pain appears complex, often ambiguous, and highly varied. Themes that emerge from the reflections of study participants on the relationship between work and the experience of pain include the prototypical American associations of work stress leading to the amplification of pain and, less frequently, pain leading to lost work days, lessened productivity, and irritability with co-workers. However, three recurrent and focal themes about the significance and meaning of work are salient in the narratives of many of the working women and men interviewed during this study, and they diverge from our culture's prototypical "work-stress-pain" theme. I characterize these themes as (1) work as a *haven* from pain and loss, (2) work as an arena for self-realization and effective performance, and (3) work as a vehicle for control over the intrusiveness and daily disruptiveness of pain.

Framing the analysis in this fashion suggests a somewhat different emphasis from that of the classical literature on chronic pain and work, much of which emphasizes the tedium or stresses of work, especially when workers lack control over their activities and environment, and the role of work in producing disability and in amplifying pain (Osterweis et al. 1987; Karasek and Theorell 1990). It also provides an interpretation of the relationship of work to chronic pain that differs from the interpretation found in both the popular writing and research associated with studies of disabled Americans. In this chapter, I wish to argue that work may at times be perceived by those who suffer from chronic pain as a palliative, an analgesic, a way to fend off or escape pain, and a way to maintain self-efficacy and achieve self-realization in spite of chronic pain. This approach is not meant to dismiss the findings of previous research, which identify the relationship between noxious dimensions of work and occupational hazards and ill health; it is rather an effort to broaden our interpretation in understanding the diverse meanings of work in the lives of those who experience chronic pain.

Our research interviews with chronic pain sufferers suggest that work often may be an active process of meaning-making and of self-constitution, especially in the face of what B. Good refers to as the "world-threatening" or "unmaking" dimensions of pain (see chap. 2). The research interviews also raise questions about conceptualizations central to one of the knotty problems of medical sociology, and more recently, of medical anthropology: What does work mean? What is its relationship to illness and to gender? How does the relationship between health and work vary by class and types of work? How do we understand these relationships? In this chapter, I briefly review literature on the diverse meanings of work in American culture and examine the research literature on the relationship of work, health, and gender. I develop my analysis with accounts from two professional working women who experience chronic pain, and I suggest the implications of a research model that focuses on the "meaning-making" dimensions of work in relationship to health and illness.

WORK AND MEANING IN AMERICAN CULTURE

For individuals who define "life as career,"[2] the significance of work is weighty, a central part of everyday experience, and it is this centrality of work which expands the boundaries of interpretation regarding the relationship between pain and work. Although this chapter focuses on the lives of professional working women, the themes presented are not meant to be limited to professionals nor to women. The centrality of work to Americans, in definition of self, in linking self to community through a "calling," through activity for the common good (Bellah et al. 1985), and through the joining of instrumental and affective expression (Smelser 1980), has been a dominant theme in the more optimistic analyses of American society and culture. Kohn (1980:205) proposes that in industrial society, work directly affects individuals' values and orientation to the world around them, what he terms the "I do, therefore I am" notion of self. This view of the self is popularly conveyed in Terkel's *Working* (1972): through presentation of narratives of working Americans, he portrays work as the search "for daily meaning as well as daily bread" (1972:xiii) and describes not only its limitations on the human spirit but the opportunity work provides for immortality, to "do something on this earth" (1972:xxx). Rubin, in *Worlds of Pain* (1976), highlights the meaning of work for the American working class and the sense of mastery and competence that is experienced by skilled laborers, women as well as men, in contrast to the stress of major work instability. Ratcliff and Bogdan (1988), in analyzing the meaning of work for women, note recent research that identifies work as a major source of satisfaction, sense of self-control, and empowerment for women, regardless of job status.

Work, Gender, and Health

Much research over the past decade in the area of gender, health, and work has attempted to address the apparent differences in health status between men and women and, in a subtle fashion, to grapple with the clinical and epidemiological model of the "somatizing" housebound woman (Brown and Harris 1978). This recent work in medical sociology suggests that for women, work outside the home of any sort, but in particular professional work, contributes to mental and physical health. Research on the relationship between gender and health has documented that women have higher physical and psychiatric morbidity than do men and are more likely to seek health care for experienced symptoms (Weissman 1977; Kessler et al. 1981; Verbrugge 1983, 1985). However, Rosenfield (1980) found that married women who worked and who had husbands who worked had lower levels of depressive symptoms than did married men whose wives worked and married women who did not work. The psychiatric symptom scores for this group of women in "non-traditional" roles were comparable to that of the total male sample. Verbrugge (1983) found that in a sample of Detroit adults, employment (as well as marriage and parenthood) for women as for men was associated with lower rates of acute and chronic diseases, lower rates of restricted-activity days and health-care visits, and lower rates of psychotropic drug use. These researchers suggest that diverse social roles that demand activity, such as work, may act as buffers against physical ill health and psychiatric morbidity, reducing risks and lowering sensitivity to symptoms. (See also Nathanson 1980; Aneshensel et al. 1981; Gore and Mangione 1983; Verbrugge 1989.) The researchers in this tradition hypothesize that women who work, especially those who have positions of high occupational control (Rosenfield 1989), not only may be empowered in their experience of competence and self-esteem, but this sense of empowerment leads to lower susceptibility to physical and psychiatric morbidity because of their diverse roles and high control activity. The relationship between social-causation models (e.g., social roles influence health) and social-selection models (e.g., health influences the number and types of roles assumed) has been less clearly worked out in the social epidemiological literature, although previous findings that women who do not work outside the home have poorer health suggest the value of both perspectives (Brown and Harris 1978; Gove and Geerken 1977; Haw 1982).[3]

Recent research in the medical anthropological literature on women and work has largely focused on working-class women and on factory and piece-work, over which one has limited control. The noxious effects of such work are identified as producing bodily and psychological distress, and as Lock argues, this bodily distress may be viewed as a mode of resistance and of protest (Lock 1990; Ong 1987). This analytic approach contrasts strikingly with the diagnostic categories of "somatization" generated in part by clinical medicine and research psychiatry (DSM-III-R).

The problem of trying to ferret out the relationship of work, gender, and health or pain poses a challenge, suggesting an extension of efforts to understand how women experience work in relationship to health. This places the meaning of work as more central to the understanding of women's integrated experience of health and illness than many of our culture's popular *historical* conceptions about women's work would suggest. Epstein, writing in the 1970s, identified American culture's view that women's work was *less* "central to women's lives, as an avenue for self-expression and stimulation" than for men (Epstein 1970); that it was but "supplementary and contingent" for middle-class women (Epstein 1970), or "stressful" for professional women because of career barriers and male dominance, resistance and antagonism (Lorber 1984; Epstein 1981). The meaning of work for the two women whose cases I have chosen to analyze for this essay stands in contrast to these traditional popular images of the meaning of work for women. These case accounts, by acknowledging the centrality of work, are intended to explore the dimensions of self-realization and meaning-making that work has for many middle-class and professional women, a feature of women's lives brought into focus by the feminist activities and research of the past two decades.[4] In addition, the analysis of these two cases seeks to extend the social epidemiological research through anthropological methods, in an effort to unmask the varieties of meaning and the ways in which women experience work in relationship to their health. These cases suggest that work may indeed act as a buffer against the amplification of chronic pain, both physical and psychiatric. Although work may be a source of dissatisfaction or stress at times and thus impact negatively on health status (Haynes and Feinlieb 1980; Cleary and Mechanic 1983; House et al. 1986; Lennon 1987), it also may act to circumscribe the centrality of pain and psychic distress in daily living. How does this happen?

Chronic Pain and Work

The case material I describe in this chapter focuses on two women, both in their early sixties, who are in highly responsible professional positions and who devote their efforts to organizations in the service of others.[5] I interviewed each of these women four times over the course of fifteen months, through a series of guided discussions; each interview lasted over ninety minutes (see note 1 for a fuller description of the project and method).

The material presented in these cases draws on the women's narrative elucidation of their experience of pain over the course of their life and their discussions about work, which emerged as centrally important not only to their self-identity but also to their experience of pain. These two women define their work as efforts to contribute to the common good of the communities in which they live and practice. Both women work with numerous people, above and below them in the hierarchy of their organizations, and their work affects the lives of hundreds of youth and children.

My analysis of each case aims to unpack the meaning that work has in the lives of these individuals, in particular as it relates to their experiences of chronic pain. Both women turn to work for self-realization and to define themselves within broader communities of persons and institutions to be served, and yet, both women experience pain daily and take nonnarcotic medications daily to dampen their pain. Throughout the interviews, work and pain emerged as essentially contrasting domains. On one hand, work was conceived by these women as a realm of meaning-making, as the central creative process and activity of their lives. Pain, on the other hand, condensed losses, unrealized goals, disappointments, and lack of control, and represented what Garro (chap. 5) has characterized as an ontological assault. Although these women are of course not representative of all working women, the cases suggest an important positive role of work for women in the constitution of the self in the face of chronic pain.

WORK AS A HAVEN FROM PAIN AND LOSS: THE CASE OF MRS. ABLE

Some work diffuses into my home life, but in a positive sense; it is not a burden. . . . I work to smooth relationships . . . to prevent conflict between the trustees and (the clients).

Going to work, that is when I have no trouble concentrating. There are wonderful times; my mind is diverted. At home, other distractible thoughts start taking over.

In fact, it almost makes me believe in fate, a forty-five-year-old woman getting an M.A., working for the first time, at real work. Progressing in a job, gaining respect. Until then, I did not even know what a "professional" was. I did not know, it was not a choice but . . . it became a whole new life for me.

Mrs. Able, aged sixty and married for almost forty years, is remarkably engaging and mentally energetic. When we first met in my office, she appeared compact, a small woman, neither lean nor heavy, although like many American women her age, she lamented her weight and complained of being in "not very good shape." Mrs. Able told me she suffers from chronic back pain and arthritic pain in her legs and joints, for which she takes eight to ten aspirin daily and an occasional five-milligram Valium at night to ease her sleep and aid in muscle relaxation. Although her pain was often not obvious, it emerged that she endured extremely serious, ongoing pain. In spite of daily discomfort, Mrs. Able works full-time, as a senior professional administrator, after progressing through the ranks of her institution over the past fifteen years. She is pleased with her educational achievements, "three degrees received in middle age," which led to her professional development. She told me several times, as she recounted the past fifteen years and how they led her to occupy her current position, that "it almost makes me believe in fate, that a forty-five-year-old woman could progress so in a profession that I did not even know existed in my younger days." The pleasure of daily work comes, she said, "from the possibility of learning more," "the people I come into contact with," "the positive responses and feelings that come from many of those I work with," and the sheer satisfaction of quenching her intellectual interests associated with her career.

As we reviewed together the impact of chronic pain on daily work schedules, Mrs. Able noted she had not missed more than one day of work in six months, that she usually works approximately forty-five hours per week and brings work home regularly, which she perceives as not a burden but rather a positive activity. Similar to many other professionals, Mrs. Able feels that she is "productive but could do more," could "be more successful" at what she does do, and that in part these limitations on her degree of success have to do with the structure of the organization in which she works and the relationship between older professional women and younger professional men. Nevertheless, Mrs. Able enjoys her work and the approval and "respect" of her colleagues, bosses, and subordinates. The "whole new life" that is represented by her current position and the achievements and activity it took to gain this position are placed against a series of personal and family traumas that are deeply associated with her experience of chronic pain. Work is clearly an arena in in which Mrs. Able experiences self-esteem and expresses competence. How, then, does she relate her work to her experience of chronic pain and to these traumas?

The Experience of Pain

Mrs. Able's experience of back pain began two decades ago; arthritic pain in her legs and joints began to be particularly bothersome one decade ago. Pain-free periods are rare, and she found that "the near daily experience of pain all but obliterates memories of pain-free periods that do occur." In the past decade, she had two auto accidents that she feels exacerbated her musculoskeletal discomfort. In 1977, she underwent surgery for colon cancer and recovered from this major illness.

Mrs. Able, like many of the study participants, characterized her overall health in a curiously mixed fashion, of healthy/not healthy. She told me in response to my question of how she considered her health—good, fair, or poor—"I think of myself generally as a healthy person, until I start to itemize my problems; I actually feel it is only fair, but it is probably good. In objective tests, my movement is good. But it is the quality I'm concerned about, the quality of my time." She attributes her musculoskeletal discomfort and pain to a deterioration of her spine and vertebrae, which she images, in reflecting on her X rays, as "crumbling, like ashes, or crumbling stone." She remarked that she did not identify the onset of her back pain with any particular event or situation, that "I assume that is what happens to people. It starts by the age of twenty-five; everybody has it (arthritis) and there is nothing to do about it." Her fears about the implication of her pain are that she will become "unable to do things, get around, take care of myself, have some fun"; she fears "being dependent and being alone."

Mrs. Able remarked, when we were talking about the constancy of pain, that the worst thing about it was "that when in pain, it is hard to remember there are times when I don't experience pain." Her image of the future course of her arthritic and back pain is rather bleak, as going "from bad to worse, hopefully with some respites." At our initial interview, when she rated her current experience of pain as mild (one on a five-point scale of the McGill Pain Questionnaire), she chose from the McGill list adjectives such as "pinching," "pulling," "aching," "tiring," "grueling," "penetrating," and "nagging" to describe her current pain. For pain experienced in the previous seven days, she added more intense descriptives, such as "wretched," "unbearable," "penetrating," "tearing," and "torturing." "Exhausting," "frightful," "lancinating," and "lacerating" were descriptives chosen in subsequent interviews along with the previous adjectives. Although such adjectives were elicited through a formal questionnaire, she engaged in the choice with intense seriousness, remarking at how one or the other fit her experience. Physical activity, such as standing, walking, or climbing steps, increases the severity of her pain. Hot baths, medication, and a glass of wine

contribute to relief of pain. Mrs. Able labeled her pain at its worst as "excruciating."

Although Mrs. Able felt that pain was a companion to physical activities,
such as walking or climbing, she remains active in professional organizations, takes a leadership role in her professional community, and gives
speeches to other women with similar career interests. She also travels, often
with colleagues, to foreign lands and engages the world. However, Mrs.
Able's satisfying interactions occur in her professional and social life away
from home and largely away from her family. She notes that one of the consequences of daily pain is a growing feeling of being alienated from her home,
of not being able to entertain at home, because of the inability to "do anything" around the house. She laments that "I accomplish very little outside
of work, and don't feel very good about that."

Several times during the course of study, I asked Mrs. Able to assess how
pain infringed upon work and vice versa, whether pain intruded on her work
accomplishments as it did in her home life. Mrs. Able felt that she works as
much and as well as others with similar positions, that she never takes "frequent rests" because of her pain, but that she does make some adjustments
(sitting, walking) in her job to accommodate her pain. She noted that she got
along well with others "most of the time," although occasionally she found
herself being irritable at work because of her pain. In our guided interviews,
when we discussed her responses to these closed questions, she commented
that she felt that even though her pain was potentially intrusive in its daily
presence, that at work in contrast to at home "I hope I have control over the
pain part." Throughout the course of our relationship, she often reflected
that she was successful in controlling pain in her work setting. This control is
strikingly evident when she contrasts it with her experiences outside of work,
in the health-care system,[6] at home, and with her family.

Mrs. Able told me several times that she had "started a whole new life" at
age forty-five, and that her current work represented this new life. Intertwined with her rather dry account of coping with chronic physical pain that
is ever expanding into her daily experience, and with her story of professional
success, couched in language suggesting considerable amazement of who she
has become as a professional, is an emotionally laden set of associations with
two major family traumas, the loss of her son and the illness of her daughter,
and the loss of a positive family future. In her reflections on her past life,
these traumas are at times loosely associated with her mid-life career development; at other times her discourse on work almost suggests that these
traumas precipitated her into a new "professional" life, not by planning or
choice but "perhaps by some grand non-human design." The issue of control
surfaces explicitly from time to time in Mrs. Able's reflections, less often with
regard to interactions at work, but frequently in relationship to her life world
beyond the domain of work.

Private Losses, Public Pain

Let me bury my dead. . . . It is as if I am living out Eugene O'Neill's *Long Day's Journey Into Night.*

I *had* a son—that's a very complex and complicated story. He would be thirty-nine on Monday. When I say we lost him, I'm not using an euphemism. He has literally been lost since 1966 and he could be anywhere, on the go, alive or dead. And I don't know . . .

The big problem I had was never being allowed to grieve. My best friend, my sister, would change the subject. My neighbors wouldn't say anything. His existence was not being acknowledged.

One of the things I regret, and I don't know if there is a way to recapture it, I don't remember my Mother. . . . There's one picture we had of her and I assume she looked like that. . . . I could never bring her face up before me except for that picture. No one ever talked to me about that—not ever. . . . Maybe that is why I reacted so strongly to people ignoring my son after he disappeared, because it is *important* for me to remember him.

Mrs. Able lost her mother when she was nine years old. She grew up in an immigrant Eastern European family that she experienced as having had no capacity to help her understand the loss of her mother. In her view, her craftsman father was untalkative; she recalled that as a child she was embarrassed that he was not a citizen and was illiterate in English. When evoking the sense of loneliness and emptiness of a motherless childhood, she recalled how as a young girl, she "never told a soul" of the onset of her menses, although she was confused by the blood, the pain, the frequency. She characterized not only her father but also her older siblings as "uncommunicative" and distant.

Married life brought middle-class status, a solid marital relationship with a spouse who was bright and "knew so much about so many things," successful pregnancies—"I never felt better in my life than when I was pregnant"—two creative children, and community involvement. When the children became adolescents, family difficulties, perhaps an articulation of American cultural movements of the era, began to erupt. She recalls interactions with school psychologists in the early sixties, and with other parents concerned about their children, with a certain bitterness, particularly about the dominant professional models of family psychology of the period. "We were a generation of parents who were labeled *vipers.* We were the enemy, and don't think that doesn't get across to your kid."

Two parallel traumas to the family occurred when the children were in their late and middle teens. Mrs. Able's son disappeared during his hitchhiking tour of the country, while on leave from college. Her daughter, several years younger, attempted suicide shortly after her brother's disappearance and began a series of psychotherapeutic treatments and hospitalizations which drained the family emotionally and economically. Her daughter's psychiatric illness is perceived by Mrs. Able as "being directly related to the loss of her brother."

This family trauma was intensified by what Mrs. Able evocatively characterized as a madness-making *limbo*, a limbo into which both she and her husband were forced, not knowing the whereabouts and situation of their son, not being consulted and confided in by their daughter's therapists. Mrs. Able considered that the destruction of these parent-child relationships was gravely injurious to both herself and her husband. Therapists appeared as hostile parties. Mrs. Able recalls one psychologist's comment about her son's disappearance—"No wonder your son ran away!"— with intense bitterness, particularly because her son did not "run away." In our interviews, she recalled with grievous sadness that the sense of being "enemy parents" was additionally exacerbated and reinforced by her daughter's psychiatrists "who deigned to speak to us." Mrs. Able's account of these events conveys how both her and her husband's sense of efficacy and control over their world was critically assaulted and permanently compromised.

It was during the years of this assault on Mrs. Able's family life that she "started a whole new life." During this period, she was in school working toward the first of her three degrees; several years after the disappearance of her son, she took her first professional position. She characterizes this time as a period of extraordinary uncertainty, of endless "not knowing," a time of hired private investigators and constant contact with the police, in what led eventually to a futile effort to find their son, "who just literally disappeared." Although the police found human remains eighteen months after her son's disappearance in approximately the last locale from which he had written to them, a positive identification could not be made.

It was also during this time of family assault, Mrs. Able told me, that she "needed to have a rationalization to stay away from home," that she was "out of the dumps only when in school," that "as far as my home is concerned, I was definitely as depressed as one can be." First school, then her professional career, came to be the focus of her efficacious life, the part of her life through which she could remake her world.

Experience and Resolution of Grief

Intellectually I think he is dead; it's been a long time. But I don't act like it.

Years of experiencing unresolved grief, of being unable even to hold the rituals to bury her dead because of religious and legal proscriptions, paralleled Mrs. Able's professional development and advancement at work. Mrs. Able, in our interviews, did not explicitly associate her health afflictions of late middle age in any direct fashion with the life traumas and losses experienced. However, when she reflects on her emotional state, her language is poignant and richly evocative, and her associations of psychic distress with emotional loss are detailed and dense.[7] Mrs. Able characterizes herself as experiencing

> a certain amount of depression all the time. It is so much of a part of me, it's just there. I cannot envision a future that has anything worth looking forward to. People ask "how can you bear it?" *What are the alternatives!* Having ruled out suicide, the way things are now . . .

> I feel no control over the important things in life. It's given, it's there (the depression, the sense of no control). . . . Do what you think you have to do.

She remarks that she thinks about suicide, about death, "that I never expected to be sixty," but feels she does not have control over her death. She contrasts her "baseline" feelings of depression with her means of coping. "At times I have more feelings of energy. People say, 'I can't keep up with you,' but that is not real, not an accurate perception on their part." Although she dismisses this channeling of energy "from irritable pacing to doing something" as not "really real," she frequently told me that she equates "feeling better" with "doing something." The "doing something" often involves helping other people, to distract oneself from one's own pain.

> I am easily distracted, I can give other people's feelings precedence over my own feelings. I don't talk about myself, reveal myself. I can dispense advice, very freely. I can get people to talk about themselves.

It is this facility that Mrs. Able has managed to incorporate into her professional work "at smoothing relationships" and attending to the needs of others.

When I interviewed Mrs. Able during our second visit, following the psychiatric interview schedule for affective disorders (a modified SADS-L), it was evident that she did not meet the research criteria for major depressive disorder. However, her marginal symptom levels were suggestive of dysthymic disorder (a low-level chronic depression). The life experiences of severe, intense, and unresolved grief, most seriously experienced over the disappearance of her son but also felt for her mother's early death (and in a sense for herself), her daughter, and her family's lost future, readily contribute to these symptom levels, to what she characterized as the experience of a "certain amount of depression all the time." When we spoke of her younger brother's recent death by heart disease, she reflected on the associations that were brought up for her anew. "I did a lot of mothering of him; he was three years old when my mother died. I found myself thinking about my brother and my son together, especially when my younger brother died." Three years ago, after numerous unsuccessful attempts at therapy for grief for her son, Mrs. Able finally found a therapist who could work with her in a meaningful way, who helped her cope not only with her brother's death but also with the unresolved grief she held for her son. It was through these successive sessions and additional follow-ups over the period of the past several years that she came increasingly able "to bury my dead."

After more recent participation in a therapeutic group, Mrs. Able recalled how the process brought into awareness for her "the anger I was still carrying toward my mother. . .for having died and left me. I was acutely sensitive to having no mother, when I married, when I had babies." The therapeutic process and several previous therapy sessions enabled Mrs. Able to not only finally "bury my dead," but to grieve over lost parents, children, siblings, and the future, which "appeared bleak." She recalled to me that while she still harbored anger at her mother ("I am a textbook case") during the group therapy, that she held no anger for her son.

> If he walked in tomorrow, I would be furious and overjoyed. I can't say "I wish he had never been born." Or ask, "Why me?" My own theology when I was growing up was almost Puritanical—you get what you deserve. I don't feel that way now. If I got what I deserve by his disappearance, I didn't deserve to live, I would have to be that bad.

Anger, unresolved grief, distress over her daughter's intractable illness, and dismay over the family's future financial as well as spiritual health would clearly unmake the world for many individuals. However, Mrs. Able has been remarkably resilient and personally effective. She speaks of this unwelcomed "fate" of family trauma as quite astonishingly opening her path toward a professional career. Such an account carries with it an intimation that this career was to be her palliative, to enable her to live with grief, disappointment, and pain.

What is intriguing about the meaning of work and of pain for Mrs. Able is that in her public life she is comfortable with her profession and views herself as very competent. In her narrative and responses to formal questions on work, she relates the normal stresses and hassles of high-powered professional work only marginally to her pain, with her pain influencing situations at work (increasing irritability), but not in turn being amplified by work-related hassles. Indeed, work as well as previous academic achievements and volunteer community activities are sources of pride, satisfaction, and at times "wonderful" diversions from troubling thoughts. In my analysis of over ten hours of interviews I conducted with Mrs. Able, it becomes evident that *work is a haven from pain*, both physical and psychological, and from intense and serious losses.

In the domain of work, Mrs. Able feels effective and, in most situations, in control. However, work also symbolizes the paradox of being in control and being effective while still subject to the vicissitudes of life. Mrs. Able finds herself musing that her larger life situation, her husband's dependency on her steady income and her central role as bread-winner, means that in certain respects she does not have control over whether she works or not. As she noted, family circumstances have meant that she cannot say "take this job and shove it" on those days when dissatisfaction is intense. Thus, although work is a haven from pain and loss and a critical source of self-realization and effectiveness, the grander scheme of things appears to wrench control and options from her.

WORK AS AN ARENA FOR REALIZING IDEALS AND COMBATTING THE INTRUSIVENESS OF PAIN: THE CASE OF MS. GRAHAM

> The human condition both saddens me and challenges me. . . . A saviour com-
> plex is what brings people into this field and keeps us going. We fix people, we
> fix situations, make things right. The human encounter bits make the work
> even more challenging. . . .
> What drives me is the wish to do a good job, to be on top of things. I choose
> not to just work nine to five. Is that driven? It is my value system, the ethics of
> my profession. . . . So is that being driven? It is to some extent. I can see a lot of
> people saying "what the hell," but not *good* people in my field.

Ms. Graham, a sixty-year-old clinician by training, is passionate about her work and her devotion to the "neglected, the abused, the emotionally disturbed." Like Mrs. Able, Ms. Graham is a high-level professional administrator in an organization devoted to community concerns, where, as she frequently noted, she "wears two hats" as a boss and as a clinician. These two roles, the instrumental "goal- and task-oriented" administrator and the affectively sensitive clinician, which she labels as "Yankee" and "not-Yankee," appear as expressions of two aspects of Ms. Graham's concept of herself, of her being, feeling and acting in her world of work. These two facets of self-identity, and the semantic domains implied, structure her discourse on the relationship of work, interpersonal life, personal history, affective state, and pain.

The Experience of Pain

Ms. Graham has experienced daily headaches and occasional severe migraines for forty years, and although unable to completely eliminate the pain, she attempts to control the intensity and intrusiveness with ten to twelve tablets of buffered aspirin or Tylenol a day. She recalls no pain-free periods in many years, but dismissing her headaches, she exclaims, "I will not let them interfere with my work! . . . I simply don't let my headaches interfere with me. Maybe one time a year will I lay my head on a bed." Ms. Graham works fifty to sixty hours per week and she chooses to "play hard," to engage in active sports—skiing, swimming, sailing, gardening—in spite of her daily headache pain.

Ms. Graham described her headaches to me as being, at their very worst, "like a jackhammer . . . a handball being played in my head . . . a hot poker in the eyes." Her vision becomes affected, with "Disney's *Fantasia*-like colored spots on a black field" whirling in front of her eyes; her equilibrium and ability to focus is also disturbed. She experiences cold sweats and the sensation of a "band of tension tied around my head." In identifying adjectives (from the McGill Pain Questionnaire) that describe her current headache pain at our first interview, she chose "beating," "pressing," "aching," "penetrating," "tight," and "intense." Similar adjectives, including "sharp" and "drilling," were selected on follow-up interviews. She labeled her headache pain as "excruciating" at its worst, but at the time of the interviews noted it was more mildly "distressing."

Commenting that "I will always have headaches . . . it is part of adult life," Ms. Graham told me she is no longer worried about the underlying meaning of her symptoms of pain. "It's been with me too long . . . historically I've gone through it." When speaking of past fears, she recalled that until approximately ten years ago, she feared she might be suffering from a brain tumor, and that "there was to be no relief from the constant and worst of the [pain]." Now she finds that she no longer has these fantasies and fears; "I know what I have and the 'worst of the predictions,' the brain tumor, has not happened: time heals all."

The reframing of headache symptoms into a medical "problem" occurred when Ms. Graham joined a health maintenance organization; during the course of initial workup and medical history, she was referred for a series of unsuccessful neurological consults. Recalling the side effects of suggested medications for combating her intermittent migraines, she noted, "Physicians have a problem with my headaches. . . . I don't present it as a problem, I haven't said 'do something.'"

Ms. Graham initially responded to my questions about her perception of underlying causes of her headaches as "not within my conscious knowledge," although she noted that severity of symptoms was associated with city pollution, allergies, and tension; that she gained relief from severity when she was in the country and active in outdoor sports. However, shortly after being asked about "causes" of pain, she recounted a powerful and moving story of childhood illness.

Recollections of Childhood and Illness

When Ms. Graham was three years old, an ophthalmologist told her parents that she would be blind before she "was out of her teens." She was extremely nearsighted as a child, wore glasses from the age of three, and was constantly restricted in her use of her vision. She was taken to physicians every six months, to "the good doctors" in her parents' best judgment. She was forbidden to read for eight years, from first grade to the first year of high school, when her diagnosis was revised. These early childhood years of serious fear of blindness coincided with parental messages that Ms. Graham labels her "task- and goal-oriented family culture." She noted that she was "conditioned from the womb . . . to go for it!" Despite her physical handicap, it was expected that she, like her healthy sibling, would achieve. Although she noted that her parents "were not inattentive" to her physical needs, she identified them both as "creators, doers, movers," who instilled in her a drive for educational attainment that overrode the "problem of reading." She was read to through elementary school; at age fourteen she was sent off to prep school and had to begin to cope with the need to read herself.

Through the course of our interviews on family and personal history, work, and psychological status, Ms. Graham recounted additional critical events during her early childhood years. Although she perceived these early childhood experiences as influencing her personality and her values about work, as well as her intermittent psychological malaise, she did not connect these experiences to her childhood illness (her restricted vision) nor to her chronic pain. Her father, whom she adored, was a scientist working for the military, often based away from home; his presence in the family during her early childhood years was irregular. When Ms. Graham was two to three years old, and again at age five, she was cared for by her paternal aunts, "while my mother was off getting cured in the hills of Pennsylvania" for tuberculosis. She recalls that the first person she remembered was not her mother but her father's sister. Her close relationship to her father's sisters was disrupted upon her mother's return home, as her mother "did not like my aunts" and "aborted" frequent contact. Ms. Graham identifies these two early separations from her mother, her father's long absences, and the distancing relationship with her aunts, as contributing to what she labels "problems of separation." She noted that her discomfort in going to prep school was in part related to fears aroused by these early experiences with separation as well as by concerns of "making it" in school, of gaining self-confidence. Self-confidence emerged with young adulthood, with success at establishing a professional career and a network of intensely satisfying friendships, at considerable distance from parental home and family.

Being "Yankee" and "Not-Yankee"

Ms. Graham's family heritage is truly "old-American": her ancestors came to America on the Mayflower. She uses her ethnicity in an intriguing way, to delineate perceived sources of her self-identity that are complementary and contradictory. Even though she is "old-American" through both maternal and paternal lineages, she plays off the "Yankee"/"not-Yankee" imagery. Although Ms. Graham does not associate her early childhood vision problems and her intermittent separation from her parents with the emergence of chronic headache pain, she does view her response to daily pain as reflective of her family's culture, which diminished the centrality of health concerns and illness and emphasized the drive for achievement and "perfectionism."[8] Her childhood illness was not to interfere with her schooling and goal- and task-orientation, just as her current headaches are not to interfere with work.

Throughout our conversations together, Ms. Graham commented on how she strives to restrict the intrusion of her chronic headache pain into her daily work and public life, how she hides her pain from all but her closest friends. And yet, Ms. Graham's ambivalence over the need to suppress the significance of pain, in contrast to her desire for "TLC" in response to emotional needs as well as to pain, was also expressed during the interviews.

Her matter-of-fact discussion of the experience of chronic pain contrasts with her more emotionally laden self-analysis of who she is and how she feels. She draws a lineage of her personal characteristics and values, Yankee from her mother and aunts, not-Yankee from her father and maternal grandfather (although they, too, are ethnically Yankee).

> I'm Yankee, in that I am stoic. The Yankee posture is to carry on, in spite of whatever. I set aside *not just feelings, but FEELING lousy.* I am not going to let it interfere with my goal-orientedness. That's a New England trait, "go for it—in an unflaky way." I am not-Yankee, in that I am able to express feelings—love, sadness, happiness—in a much more open way. This is in part due to my training and in part gained from my Dad, who was a warm guy, and complemented the drivenness of my mother.

In recounting the role her family culture played in shaping her career and professional capabilities, Ms. Graham cites her parents' common Yankee values—their "common sense, clear thinking, task-oriented, strong work ethic, and intellectual values . . . their Christian ethic of integrity, honesty, setting standards, being true to oneself." She identifies her drivenness at work, her desire for perfectionism, her wish "to never make a mistake," and her need "to do things right . . . fear of not doing things right . . . fear of being criticized" to her mother's seriousness, criticalness, high expectations, and belief that life was "not meant to be enjoyed." However, she also perceives herself as gaining her competence and organizational and managerial skills from her mother as well as from her father. She identifies her clinical acumen, her ability to be an empathetic boss, her warmth and humor (which she mobilizes at work for those she supervises), her capacity for making deep friendships, and her scientific-mindedness, as inherited from her father.

These oppositions, affective and expressive versus instrumental, "warmth and humor" versus "overseriousness," clinician versus boss, not-Yankee versus Yankee, father versus mother, were salient, recurring themes in our interviews. Ms. Graham integrates the meaning of her experience of chronic pain and its relationship to her professional self and to her work through these themes. In addition, she relates these dichotomies not only to her personal characteristics but also to her current affective state and to what she identified through the course of our interviews as her "baseline depression."

Disorders of Affect: "In Public or in My Heart of Hearts?"

My moods come to the fore only when there is time for them to surface. My mood is secondary when I am getting stuff done; my self is secondary. As long as I am focusing on tasks, my concentration overrides feelings of depression. But when there is a break, then I become aware of these feelings.

My headaches are the same way, they are there all the time. And I am convinced that my mood [depression] is there all the time. The baseline never goes, it is always there. [Superficially] . . . I am in a good mood most of the time, for example when I am gardening, skiing, doing something physical, when my head is turned off, when I am most relaxed. But if you asked me if it was there, I would say yes. My experiential sense is that it is not there, but for you to ask me—it brings it into consciousness.

I am certainly different with people I know well, I share my lousy feelings. . . . But on the job, I am diplomatic. I follow the behavior code expected of me because I am a boss. I do not mask feelings, I withhold feelings except with friends. . . . I think people would be surprised to know how lousy I feel.

The manner in which Ms. Graham manages her feelings of depression and how she manages her chronic headache pain are parallel. Work and physical play serve to fend off the intrusiveness of chronic headache and psychological pain. Focused task- and goal-oriented activity are the analgesics for both modes of pain. Attention to solving the problems of others relieves her from focusing on her own pain. She interprets this process of restricting the intrusiveness of both psychological and physical pain within two meaningful frameworks; the first framework, that of her family culture, we discussed above. The second framework is largely informed by Ms. Graham's clinical knowledge and sophistication. Her interpretation of her own affective states in response to the SADS-L questions on affective disorders (see note 1) was exceptionally insightful and deep, although she has not been in psychotherapy since early adulthood, when she briefly saw a psychiatrist about complications from allergies and headache pain. Her recollection of that interaction with the medical system was strongly negative.

Ms. Graham met criteria for current and past dysthymic disorder.[9] She identifies the onset of her first episode as occurring during the last several years of boarding school, when she felt herself to be an outsider both at school and at home and was struggling academically with apparent dyslexia related to her stunted reading skills. "I never had a base, no roots, no community of peers, neither male nor female, until after college. Dad moved every eighteen months; it was an awful problem, I have never gotten over it." She attributes the chronicity of her feelings of depression to "some damn childhood thing," to "a very critical, perfectionistic mother who expected a lot," to her own self-critical qualities, her alienation from people "which was my mother's nature—I have twenty percent of it . . . I *had* eighty percent of it, but went through a whole lot of pain and struggle and behavior-moded myself out of it. I will do it until I die." She stated that she did not perceive a direct relationship between her depression and her childhood vision problems or her current chronic pain.

Ms. Graham interprets her ongoing experience of what she terms her "baseline" "fundamental depression" as arising from being self-critical, angry, wanting to be loved and valued, and fearing that is not to be. Acknowledging these feelings, she claims, is "not-Yankee." She notes that feelings of "lack of satisfaction" with her self can "create feelings of depression"; thus concern about "who I am not" leads to feeling "very lonesome and isolated." Such feelings seem not to be related to "things per se," but rather "come out of the blue, episodically." When these episodes occur, she is plagued by thoughts that "everything is terrible and I am the worst." She states that she makes "conscious use of activity to set it aside" and that "others can't tell" whether "I am positively motivated [in my activities] or fending off" feelings of depression. She thus finds activity to be "a useful and good mechanism" for getting through these most difficult periods.

The amplification of both depression and chronic pain occurred when Ms. Graham was quite senior in her career. For two years, she was waylaid in her professional work after budget restrictions decimated programs with which she was associated. She recalls these years of creating "several nutty jobs" for herself, of doing "odds and ends" to keep "as busy as I could," as a period in which her baseline depression surfaced along with greater awareness of her headache pain. During this time, for two to three years, Ms. Graham experienced symptoms that are characteristic of major depressive disorder, including vegetative and affective signs and symptoms.[10] She noted that although she did not attempt suicide, she thought of it often and was at times overwhelmed with feelings of worthlessness and the idea that "nothing was worth a damn, really." A complementary response, however, counteracted these depressive and hopeless thoughts: "I was too mad to do it; I was not going to let the world lay this on me." The Yankee "go-for-it" values surfaced intermittently, and she was able to continue her job search and to "get hold of it—take care of it," although she remarked she did not think she was directly cognizant of how seriously depressed she was at the time. Symptoms of major depression subsided on return to work, except for continuing sleep disturbance. Although Ms. Graham sought no psychiatric help during this period, she did turn to her friends for succor and assistance. She commented during the history of major depressive disorder portion of the SADS-L interview that "medical people don't suit me . . . I think I'll become a Christian Scientist."

Ms. Graham has several very good friends with whom she socializes, and she is very close to her siblings' children. Yet she still expressed occasional dismay at being a single older woman in this society. She identifies her desire to be valued not only with family and friendship relationships, which she usually finds satisfactory, but also with her work relationships. It is this relational aspect of life that in her "heart of hearts" emerges as disturbing. When feelings of depression surface, she exclaims that there is a "whole tremendous narcissistic put-upon the self," that it is then that she thinks "nobody loves me; I can't do anything right; why don't people pay attention to me?" But then, in characteristic fashion, she fends off these thoughts as not worth the time and energy. Yet it is when these feelings are at their worst that she wishes she could "sit on someone's lap, have them rock me, hold me."

Reflections on Work, Pain, Depression

Adult maturation is when you learn from your pain, from what you trip and fall on. Or at least one could. I am a very different administrator this time than I was ten years ago. It is a learning and evolutionary process.

My attitude about my headaches is no different over the last forty years. What is different in me is my need to be less driven and less perfectionistic. It is a function of talking myself out of it. I was much too angry [at failures in organizational systems] twenty years ago. Now I can set that anger aside. . . . I am mellower. My convictions haven't changed, I am mellower in how I go after them.

In our concluding interview, Ms. Graham reflected once again on the relationship of her work life to her management of chronic headache pain and baseline depression. In our discussion, she was cheerfully reflective in speaking about her work, how she *is* (very competent, a supportive administrator who takes responsibility and is valued for making decisions), and how she *would like to be* (a little lighter, more valued for her not-Yankee self). She felt that two central themes continued to weave through her work experience—that work is pleasure (her father's attitude) and that she should "do the job right in spite of one's self" (her mother's modeling). "She [my mother] was a very interesting combination of being [in chronic pain], at times very sick, but also very driven." Ms. Graham also commented on how she had posed "a question for myself: Is there a better way to deal with my fundamental depression?" Work, of course, is related to her "soul-searching," since she sees altering her behavior at work, becoming "more mellow" and less self-critical, as one way of redefining how she experiences affect.

The hopeful element in Ms. Graham's narratives, in which she weaves concerns and reflections on work, depression, and pain with her family culture and personal relationships, is her focus on maturation, "learning from one's pain," be it psychological—her overt meaning in the above comment—or physical. The dual themes through which she interprets and unpacks the meaning of both physical and psychological pain as well as the meaning of her work appear to represent the struggle within herself to come to resolution about how she wants to be during this phase of adult maturity.

It is through this struggle over meaning that Ms. Graham cognitively rede-
fines her experiences of chronic pain and depression. Work, which is the
arena in which to express both facets of herself, is central to the process of
this redefinition.

CONCLUSION

Although Mrs. Able and Ms. Graham are of different ethnic and status-
group backgrounds (Eastern European and Yankee), and although the
manner in which they express their physical pain and psychic distress is a
lesson in cultural contrast (a contained but emotional ragefulness versus a
stoic suppressed dismay), their narratives on chronic pain, work, and self
capture a common American theme, a symbolic dualism that highlights the
tension between the public world of work and the "private world" of family
and personal life.[11] If we examine the narratives of each of these women, we
find striking parallels as each constructs a divided self, a competent professional self and a personal self in physical and psychic pain. It is in the realm
of the world of work that both women experience control and a sense of
integrated selves. It is in the private world of personal and family life that
control is tenuous, life is threatening, chronic pain intrudes, and "baseline"
depression surfaces.

In reviewing Mrs. Able's account, we find a recurrent opposition between
work and family life, between that over which she can exercise control (her
pain as well as her professional achievements) and that which she fears is out
of her control (her family relationships, her grief and depression, her physical
pain). However, Mrs. Able at times regards her professional career as having
emerged from what she refers to as a "grander nonhuman design," as "fate."
In such a design, she perceives the traumas she experienced in her personal
and family history—the death of her mother, alienation from her siblings
and father, the loss of her son, and the illness of her daughter—as having
propelled her, in a fateful fashion, into this new professional life. Although
she experiences the domain of work as a haven from pain and as a locale of
control, the fact that she must work in order to maintain her family and
household is part of her fate and beyond her control.

The recurrent oppositions in Ms. Graham's narrative are more sharply
articulated (and had likely been expressed to friends prior to our interviews).
"Yankee" and "not-Yankee" not only stand for complementary aspects of
Ms. Graham's self, which she strives to integrate, but also are oppositional,
contradictory, and at times problematic aspects of the self. In our joint analysis, through the course of hours of interviews, Ms. Graham shaped her Yankee and not-Yankee self to the experience of chronic headache pain. Such
interpretations eventually entered her narrative, suggesting that in a certain
way her experience of chronic headache pain and the aggressive manner in

which she seeks to control it and "set it aside" is a manifestation of her Yankee self. In contrast, her baseline depression and her inability to overcome it are an expression of her not-Yankee self. Although she does not causally link her physical pain with her psychological depression, she readily recognized work as not only a mode of defense against both types of suffering but also the arena in which she strives to integrate her Yankee and not-Yankee approaches to restricting the intrusion of pain and depression. It is also through her work that she seeks, quite successfully, to resolve the contradictions and tensions, to right the balance of these oppositional aspects of her self.

When we examine the family histories of these two women, we find that the central traumas for each are rather remarkably mirrored and addressed in their world of professional work. Mrs. Able's source of deepest grief and depression was the loss of her son and the serious illness of her daughter, both occurring when her children entered young adulthood. Much of Mrs. Able's professional work is devoted to "smoothing relations" between older persons with power and young adults. If we reflect on Mrs. Able's recollection of therapists whose help was sought in efforts to smooth relations between parents and children, on her vivid language when she recalled therapists who labeled her generation of parents as "vipers," we might ask whether it is not through her professional work that Mrs. Able has sought to remake her world, to redress her history of family trauma and personal pain.

Ms. Graham experienced what she termed "problems of separation" in her early childhood, her experience of "never having a base, no roots, no community of peers." Part of her professional work is devoted to solving problems of child abandonment and family separation. Can it be that it is through professional work that Ms. Graham has realized and managed the source of her greatest anguish and distress as well?

Curiously, such explicit associations between choice of work and the traumatic dimensions of personal and family history were not made by either woman in our hours of interviews; as interviewer, I came to this interpretation only after reconstructing each woman's narrative.

Work as a haven from pain, physical and psychological, emerges as a vivid reality for both these women. It may be that work is a means not only to fend off the intrusion of daily pain and depression, to manipulate pain and thus make it less central in daily life, but also to conquer the essential traumas of personal life. Work therefore has the potential to be transformative as well as therapeutic.

These two cases challenge the linear models of epidemiology which have been developed to tease out and make sense of relationships between work and chronic pain or among work, gender, and health variables. When compared with other cases in the study, they remind us that work is not simply more or less stressful but that the very meaning of work has undergone important historical and generational changes in American society. These two women, both sixty years old at the onset of our interview year, were engaged in professional work they perceived to be an expression of commitment to civic or common good; work was for both a kind of "calling." For Ms. Graham, work became an expression of her family's "Yankee" culture, their drive and direction, their mastery over their environment, their commitment to the social environment within which they lived and worked. For Mrs. Able, her involvement in a professional career was part of a "grand scheme" that transcends human experience—a somewhat less controlled "fate," perhaps a less willful sense of career, a veritable "calling." Work was also the domain for each of these women in which aspects of private struggles and traumas were played out. For Mrs. Able, work was a place to exercise control and competence in the face of personal and family traumas over which she had no control. For Ms. Graham, work was the arena in which she sought to integrate, modify, balance, and bring to maturity her Yankee and not-Yankee self.

When I compare the narratives of these two women with those of five younger individuals I interviewed, I am struck with the contrast in the meaning of work as related to pain and to sense of self. These younger five—four women and a man in management, administration, or the professions—were between age twenty-eight and thirty-eight. They had quite a different sense of self and of work. In contrast to Mrs. Able and Ms. Graham, these younger individuals did not treat their careers as professions that expressed their social commitment; rather, a career was considered a way of developing the self. Although work was a path to self-realization as it was for the older women, and although it was at times talked about as a haven or a vehicle to fend off depression or pain, it was also an arena for performance and perfection of the self, thus experienced as stressful and at times related to symptoms of chronic pain or psychological distress.[12] All five of these younger people were plagued by the need to achieve "perfection." Throughout hours of interviews, themes about achieving or failing to achieve or struggling to achieve "perfection" recur. All five also incorporated the "stress" model into their narratives, associating work as well as personal stress with an exacerbation or triggering of symptoms of pain. The popularization of the "work → stress → ill health" model occurred during the course of these younger individuals' youth, when it became a dominant cultural construct. These differences may thus reflect a generational shift in the meaning of work.[13] This contrast raises a series of questions for future exploration of work and pain, suggesting an analysis that would investigate the relationship of health to cultural changes in the meaning of work in terms of self-realization and social commitment.

Future analyses of work, pain, and health, or work, gender, and health, will thus require exploring the cultural and social dimensions of how work becomes therapeutic and transformative. It will be important to examine variations in cultural constructs of work, not only for individuals and by type and institutional context of work but also by class, gender, and generation.

ACKNOWLEDGMENTS

I thank Byron Good, Arthur Kleinman, Leon Eisenberg, Paul Brodwin, and anonymous reviewers for their reading of earlier drafts of this paper and for helpful suggestions. I particularly appreciate the contribution of study participants who generously shared their thoughts and gave their time in order to convey to others the experience of chronic pain. To maintain the anonymity of participants, names have been changed and identifying details not essential to this analysis have been altered.

NOTES

1. The case material included in this chapter is from a larger study of thirty-eight patients who experienced pain for three or more months. The project was funded in part by NSF grant to Professor Arthur Kleinman, project PI. Interviews took place over the course of twelve to eighteen months, and participants were interviewed four or five times. Interview schedules included guided life history questions, as well as formal instruments, including the SADS-L, the McGill Pain Questionnaire, and a series of questions on the relationship of pain to daily functioning, including family and work life. Each interview lasted from 1 1/2 to 2 1/2 hours. Formal instruments, including the SCL-90, were completed at six-month intervals by participants. In this paper, I report on individuals I interviewed as part of this project; accounts are drawn from the series of interviews and are presented not in a single patient narrative, but rather are placed in a mosaic in an effort to convey the relationship of the experience of chronic pain and psychological distress to the meaning of work and its place in the lives of these women. Some material is drawn from taped interviews, some from notes in response to open questions, and some from the formal instruments. The individuals interviewed were currently working and none were seeking disability payments.

2. "Life as career" was the pithy comment of one of our male professionals who saw his life as equal to his work. Success in life was contingent on success in his workaday world, and book writing, for this middle-aged academic, was the key measure of his work and life success. Lillian Rubin, in *Worlds of Pain*, comments on the fusion of work time and off time, that the stress of professional work may derive from requirements of too much commitment to work (1976:190,197). This pattern, she argues, contrasts with that of the working-class families she interviewed, where work, while important to working-class men, creates problems because many working-class jobs require too little commitment of self. In contrast, she notes that working-class women who work outside the home often experience pride in "feeling competent" and in "doing a good job" and receive satisfaction from the adult world of work unattainable from the world of home (1976:168–169). Rubin argues that this

satisfaction working-class women express, even with low-paying jobs, stems from women's expressive and relational skills being utilized at work, in contrast to under-utilization in daily household chores. Rosen also captured the lives of working-class women in *Bitter Choices: Blue-Collar Women In and Out of Work*; she found that "their earnings give them increased control over the vagaries of an uncertain economic future and add to their self-esteem" (1987:168).

3. The social causation versus social selection arguments pose the question of the directional relationship between work and health. The social-causation argument, such as that emphasized by House et al. (1986) in their analysis of longitudinal data from the Tecumseh Community Health epidemiological study, identifies objective job characteristics and perceived job rewards and pressures as impacting on health behaviors, morbidity, and eventually mortality. The social-selection argument suggests that the healthy are more able to take on multiple roles, including jobs that provide greater rewards. Neither position credits sufficient importance to economic and class environments.

4. Given Rubin's findings and the findings from Verbrugge and others that employment itself may be significant for women's self-realization and sense of efficacy as well as their health status, it may be inappropriate to limit the phenomenon of work's meaning-making to the middle and professional classes or to attribute it to changes in labor and career opportunities for women in the past two decades. This raises questions as to the complexity of the meaning of alienation from work and satisfaction or independence gained from work.

5. My analysis also draws on interviews I conducted with other women in the study. I chose these two women for the focus of this essay because they had each experienced more severe and longer-lasting chronic pain than the younger women in the study and because they best illustrated the theme of work as a haven, although this theme was present for all of the younger women I interviewed as well.

6. Curiously, Mrs. Able viewed most of her diseases as integral to the process of aging, and perhaps genetic, but clearly based in biology. Thus, when Mrs. Able participated in a pain group, she expressed irritation at what she perceived was a failure of the group's physician leaders to include assessments of *biological* processes and constraints and an "automatic assumption that whatever illness we had, it was directly controllable—it doesn't take into account disease. Maybe the way you react to disease is possible to bring under control" but, she implied, the biological processes that led to physical degeneration were not.

7. Mrs. Able was not unlike other participants in the pain study in her extent of experience of family trauma and losses. Of the thirty-eight individuals in the study, 24 percent experienced either the death or disappearance of a parent, 42 percent experienced estrangement from a parent or a sibling, 34 percent had parents with major physical disabilities or chronic pain, 45 percent had parents who suffered major illnesses, and 47 percent had parents or siblings who had experienced psychological disabilities that were assessed by our participants as serious. These experiences occurred in childhood or young adulthood.

8. Certain analysts would characterize this as "denial," others "a culturally patterned response of stoicism," or "social modeling process." (See Zborowski 1969; Zola 1983; Lipton and Marbach 1984.)

9. Ms. Graham's symptoms for current and past dysthymia as elicited by the

SADS-L interview included sleep disturbance, feelings of worthlessness, tearfulness, rumination, irritability and anger at self, inability to take pleasure in praise. In addition, Ms. Graham commented that a major component of her depression is the feeling that she is unloved—"the whole tremendous narcissistic put-upon self"—and a pervasive sense of alienation.

10. Symptoms of major depression elicited by the SADS-L interview included weight loss, sleep disturbance (middle of the night awakening), loss of interest and pleasure in everything including sexual activities, alternating agitation and lethargy, feelings of guilt, trouble concentrating, and suicidal ideation.

11. In *Habits of the Heart* the symbolic dualism and tension derive from what the authors characterize as a late twentieth-century version of "individualism" and commitment to community (altogether too weak in their moral analysis); the public and competitive world of work is viewed as impoverished for many Americans as work has lost the vocational dimensions of a "calling" to labor, not solely for self-aggrandizement, but for the common and civic good. Both Mrs. Able and Ms. Graham may represent the old and lauded values that the authors wish Americans would turn to again, in that work is activity for the civic good as well as a haven from personal pain both physical and psychic.

12. Of the five cases, one man and two of the women suffered symptoms of dysthymia; one young woman suffered agoraphobia and panic disorder, which her mother had also had. She was cured during the course of the year of both her chronic headaches and her agoraphobic and panic disorder symptoms. One woman suffered from serious chronic pain in multiple sites and had a history of major depressive disorder associated with family traumas, abandonment, and alienation. Two women were high symptom attenders and did not have severe bouts of chronic pain, but one suffered intermittently from symptoms of depression.

13. Certainly older Americans frequently disparage the younger generation's linking of "work and stress," "shirking legitimate work," and using ill health caused by "stress" as an excuse to avoid work. Such comments were made by many older Americans interviewed for a study of psychosocial dimensions of primary care in rural northern California communities. The research was conducted from 1981 through 1983, with follow-up ethnographic work in 1985 and 1987, and was partially funded by NIMH grant no. MH16463 and NIMH grant no. MH39532.

REFERENCES CITED

Aneshensel, Carol S., Ralph R. Frerichs, and Virginia Clark
    1981   Family roles and sex differences in depression. *Journal of Health and Social Behavior* 22:379–393.
Bellah, Robert N., Richard Madsen, William M. Sullivan, Ann Swidler, and Steven M. Tipton
    1985   *Habits of the heart: Individualism and commitment in American life.* Berkeley, Los Angeles, London: University of California Press.
Brown, George, and Tirril Harris
    1978   *Social origins of depression: A study of psychiatric disorder in women.* New York: The Free Press.

Chapman, C. R.
  1984   New directions in the understanding and management of pain. *Social Science and Medicine* 19:639–645.
Cleary, Paul, and David Mechanic
  1983   Sex differences in psychological distress among married people. *Journal of Health and Social Behavior* 24:111–121.
Cypress, B. K.
  1983   The national ambulatory medical care survey, United States, January 1980–December 1981. Patterns of Ambulatory Care in General and Family Practice. National Center for Health Statistics, series 13, no. 73. DHHS No. (PHS) 83-1734, U.S. Government Printing Office, 1983.
Epstein, Cynthia Fuchs
  1970   *Woman's place.* Berkeley, Los Angeles, London: University of California Press.
  1981   *Women in law.* New York: Basic Books.
Good, Mary-Jo D., Byron Good, and Paul Cleary
  1987   Do patient attitudes influence physician recognition of psychosocial problems in primary care? *Journal of Family Practice* 25:53–59.
Gore, Susan, and Thomas W. Mangione
  1983   Social roles, sex roles and psychological distress: Additive and interactive models of sex differences. *Journal of Health and Social Behavior* 24:300–312.
Gove, W. R., and M. R. Geerken
  1977   The effect of children and employment on the mental health of married men and women. *Social Forces* 56:66–76.
Haw, Mary Ann
  1982   Women, work and stress: A review and agenda for the future. *Journal of Health and Social Behavior* 23:132–144.
Haynes, S. G., and M. Feinlieb
  1980   Women, work and coronary heart disease: Prospective findings from the Framingham heart study. *American Journal of Public Health* 70:133–141.
House, James S., Victor Strecher, Helen L. Metzner, and Cynthia Robbins
  1986   Occupational stress and health among men and women in the Tecumseh Community Health Study. *Journal of Health and Social Behavior* 27:62–77.
Karasek, Robert, and Tores Theorell
  1990   *Stress, productivity, and the reconstruction of working life.* New York: Basic Books.
Kessler, Ronald C., Roger L. Brown, and Clifford L. Broman
  1981   Sex differences in psychiatric help-seeking: Evidence from four large scale surveys. *Journal of Health and Social Behavior* 22:49–63.
Kessler, Ronald C., James S. House, and J. Blake Turner
  1987   Unemployment and health in a community sample. *Journal of Health and Social Behavior* 28:51–59.

Kohn, Melvin L.
  1980   Job complexity and adult personality. In *Themes of work and love in adulthood*, N. Smelser and E. Erikson, eds., 193–210. Cambridge, Mass.: Harvard University Press.
Lennon, Mary Clare
  1987   Sex differences in distress: The impact of gender and work roles. *Journal of Health and Social Behavior* 28:290–305.
Lipton, J. A., and J. J. Marbach
  1984   Ethnicity and the pain experience. *Social Science and Medicine* 19:1279–1298.
Lock, Margaret
  1990   On being ethnic: The politics of identity breaking and making in Canada, or *Nevra* on Sunday. *Culture, Medicine and Psychiatry* 14:237–254.
Lorber, Judith
  1984   *Women physicians: Careers, status and power*. New York: Tavistock Publications.
Nathanson, Constance A.
  1980   Social roles and health status among women: The significance of employment. *Social Science and Medicine* 14A:463–471.
Ong, Aihwa
  1987   *Spirits of resistance and capitalist discipline*. Albany, N.Y.: SUNY Press.
Osterweis, Marian, Arthur Kleinman, and David Mechanic
  1987   *Pain and disability*. Washington, D.C.: National Academy Press.
Ratcliff, Kathryn S., and Janet Bogdan
  1988   Unemployed women: When "social support" is not supportive. *Social Problems* 35:54–63.
Rosen, Ellen Israel
  1987   *Bitter choices: Blue-collar women in and out of work*. Chicago: University of Chicago Press.
Rosenfield, Sarah
  1980   Sex differences in depression: Do women always have higher rates? *Journal of Health and Social Behavior* 21:33–42.
  1989   The effects of women's employment: Personal control and sex differences in mental health. *Journal of Health and Social Behavior* 30:77–91.
Rubin, Lillian B.
  1976   *Worlds of pain: Life in the working-class family*. New York: Basic Books.
Smelser, Neil J., and Erik H. Erikson
  1980   *Themes of work and love in adulthood*. Cambridge, Mass.: Harvard University Press.
Terkel, Studs
  1972   *Working*. New York: Viking Penguin.
Verbrugge, Lois
  1983   Multiple roles and physical health of women and men. *Journal of Health and Social Behavior* 24:16–29.

1985   Gender and health: An update on hypotheses and evidence. *Journal of Health and Social Behavior* 26:156–182.
1989   The twain meet: Empirical explanations of sex differences in health and mortality. *Journal of Health and Social Behavior* 30:282–304.

Weissman, Myrna, and Gerald Klerman
1977   Sex differences and the epidemiology of depression. *Archives of General Psychiatry* 34:98–111.

Zborowski, Mark
1969   *People in pain.* San Francisco: Jossey-Bass.

Zola, Irving K.
1983   Culture and symptoms: An analysis of patients' presenting complaints. In *Socio-medical inquires*, 86–108. Philadelphia: Temple University Press.

CHAPTER FOUR

Symptoms and Social Performances: The Case of Diane Reden[1]

Paul E. Brodwin

The talk of people with chronic pain is filled with vivid metaphors. A man with lower back pain reports that his spine "is being split apart"; a woman describes a debilitating pain in her shoulders as "a big lump—red and hot— of muscles, nerves, tendons bunched together" (Kleinman 1988). These striking images derive their power from the metaphoric use of language. They reveal the creative ability of certain people to convey a visceral sense of their suffering through a well-chosen phrase. They represent one way, and perhaps the most powerful way, to express through a common language the private and wordless reality of chronic physical pain. But they also suggest a much larger theme, which this chapter will examine in detail: the ways in which pain exhibits some of the qualities of a human language.

This chapter tells the story of Diane Reden, a young woman with a dizzying array of mutable and seemingly uncontrolled pain symptoms. Diane relies on her body and its sufferings to communicate with and influence the people around her. Her pain symptoms function like a language, and this perspective on her suffering catches something that is missed by the more common conceptual frameworks from psychology or psychiatry. Since the chapter will employ several terms—metaphor, rhetoric, and performance —not usually found in case studies of chronic illness, some initial definitions are in order.

When someone with ulcerative colitis reports his stomach "is tied up in knots" or a migraine sufferer says her head feels like "it's made out of glass," they are using language in a figurative way. In particular, these expressions work as *metaphors*: they transpose meaning between two radically different domains. In one instance, a man's private but unmistakable sensation of abdominal pain is symbolically connected to the visual image of a (perhaps hopelessly) tangled rope. In the other instance, a woman's bodily experience of extreme vulnerability to noise and light is connected to the image of a fragile glass sphere, easily broken and needing special protection from its surroundings.

Such metaphors exemplify the nonliteral use of language. Although they point to an immediate physical experience, they do not establish a simple correspondence between words and an objective physical reality. In any other context, ropes and stomachs or headaches and thin glass spheres have nothing whatsoever in common. But when persons in pain invoke these incongruous images, they actually endow their pain with new meanings. The use of metaphor creatively restructures both the experience of chronic pain as well as its place in a person's most important social relations. To understand this process takes us to a related area: the rhetoric of chronic pain.

Both the talk about pain and even the bodily symptoms themselves can express certain emotions and desires, deliberately directed at an audience to convince them to act a certain way. They can have a demonstrable effect in a person's local social world; this exemplifies the rhetorical aspect of chronic pain. By drawing attention to a particular set of symptoms (or by visibly and dramatically suffering from them), one can avoid unpleasant activities or gain extra support. For example, the husband whose chronic backache suddenly worsens the day before a planned visit to a disliked in-law (Kotarba 1983) exemplifies the interpersonal use of this rhetoric. It can also be used in the workplace (especially when pain complaints are the only legitimate excuse for time off or reduced work loads) and within the family (as will be outlined in Diane Reden's case).

A vast psychological literature on chronic pain focuses precisely on such "secondary gains" (see Fordyce 1976; Turk et al. 1983; Holzman and Turk 1986). Much of this research, building on a behaviorist paradigm, focuses on the pathological effects of chronic pain upon family functioning, for example, the manipulative "pain games" of patients who use their symptoms to dominate other family members or escape responsibilities (Menges 1981). However, viewing such symptoms primarily as rhetoric allows a broader (and perhaps less judgmental) interpretation. This rhetoric helps chronic pain sufferers communicate their wants and needs in crucial social relationships, especially when the use of other languages is not sanctioned.

The rhetoric of pain can become stabilized as the dominant medium of communication in certain local settings: a community, a clinic, or even a family. For example, Minuchin and his colleagues (Minuchin et al. 1978) have examined the family factors accompanying children's disorders (diabetes, asthma, and especially anorexia nervosa). They claim that the interpersonal transactions among family members sustain many psychosomatic disorders. Indeed, family interaction patterns seem to contribute as much as other mechanisms on the physiological, endocrine, or biochemical levels to produce the disease of anorexia nervosa. Such "psychosomatic families"—

characterized by enmeshment, overprotectiveness, rigidity, and lack of conflict resolution—encourage children to exemplify family conflicts through physical symptoms.

The following case study will elaborate the discussion of the metaphors of chronic pain and their rhetorical uses. The story of Diane Reden suggests the many ways in which chronic pain resembles a human language. It builds on Minuchin's insights by showing that chronic physical illness is not just the emblem of particular dysfunctional family patterns; it is also an effective idiom of communication in its own right. The case study then traces the links between Diane's unique pain symptoms and the multiple performances she faces in her daily life, and this will shed light on how the language of pain is implicated in the broader notion of "social performance."

CASE STUDY

Diane Reden's appearance is unremarkable. Dressed conservatively, looking younger than her twenty-eight years, she expresses herself hesitantly in a quiet voice that occasionally breaks, and sometimes trails off into silence in mid sentence. She is not visibly in pain—she neither grimaces, nor limps, nor touches or guards a sensitive area. But she is clearly not at ease with her body. She sits perched near the edge of her chair with a tense, vigilant expression and nervously takes long inhalations from her cigarette.

Diane's life seems unremarkable as well. Currently working as a payroll secretary in a small engineering company, Diane is single, and her social life, until recently, revolved around her family (who live nearby) and the local Catholic church. She is basically dissatisfied with her job, which she finds stupid and far below her career goals. Her social networks are both stifling and nonsupportive, but she does not plan to establish any others. A high school graduate, Diane still seems to be just starting out in life. She feels no more at ease at home, at church, with her friends, or, significantly, with herself than she did ten years ago.

Diane's medical symptoms, however, are the most remarkable aspect of her life. Painful, diverse, changeable, and seemingly uncontrollable, Diane's physical complaints include headaches, stomach pains, hyperventilation, the brief inability to see or to breathe, and many others. Unlike many pain patients, Diane does not suffer from a single overriding pain disorder, but similar to many such patients, she is engaged in a self-conscious and insightful search for the meaning of her symptoms.

In the stories that she tells about her pain, Diane uses her symptoms to represent and attempt to resolve the predicament she faces in belonging to family, church, and workplace without losing herself in them. Diane lives in a constrictive social world that seems to offer limited options for the future and a narrow range of acceptable roles for her in the present. She can see only one way of belonging to this world: meeting other people's expectations—in other words, performing for them. As this case study will demonstrate, the pain symptoms themselves represent both a performance and a protest against the demand to perform she feels within virtually all her relationships. Diane thus uses her body (and its sufferings) to communicate with and influence her social world. Her pain symptoms function like a language. Indeed, her bodily messages can speak with an authenticity and power that her verbal messages often lack.

Diane Reden has taken an indeterminate situation—vague and shifting pain symptoms in a complex web of work and family relationships—and has woven a compelling account. The case study and the interpretations that follow examine both her physical ailments and her stories about their place in her life. These interpretations of Diane's symptoms contain broader lessons for the anthropological study of chronic pain: they elucidate the twin themes of (1) pain as performance and (2) the linguistic character of pain disorders.

First of all, Diane's case illustrates how chronic pain sufferers organize their symptoms as a *performance* before different audiences (family, friends, and co-workers). For Diane, moreover, this performance threatens to generalize to other domains of her life. It can overshadow her other social roles and drive a wedge of suspicion and frustration between her and the people who comprise her several audiences. Second, Diane's story demonstrates that chronic pain symptoms communicate various messages in particular social contexts. But pain sufferers like Diane do not abandon verbal communication, nor do they necessarily lose awareness of the emotional meanings (and social uses) of their physical symptoms. Rather, they use bodily and verbal media simultaneously, and a coherent anthropological analysis must take account of both.

Description of Symptoms

Diane explains that she is never without pain; at least one of her symptoms is always present. For example, she has headaches and sinus trouble every day and migraine headaches approximately every other month. She also complains of asthma, hyperventilation, stomachaches, diarrhea, allergies, "and they even found a planter's wart on my foot." To cope with these symptoms, she takes as much aspirin as she feels she needs, often six tablets a day for weeks at a time. She also takes Triphen for her sinuses, Fiorinal for migraine headaches, and Terbutaline and Allupren (an inhaler) for her asthma. She uses a number of these drugs prophylactically. Before a headache turns into a migraine, she takes Fiorinal. At the very first sign of trouble breathing, she turns to her antiasthma medication.

Some of these symptoms have plagued Diane for most of her life, while others first appeared in her early adulthood. For example, Diane has had asthma since she was ten years old. During high school she was rushed to the hospital nearly every week in the grip of an attack. She describes these attacks: "It starts off like being short of breath, then gasping for air. Then it's like having an elastic band around my neck, preventing me from breathing." She can never quite escape from the fear of these attacks, and this fear itself produces troubling symptoms: "When I get panicky, I fear an asthma attack coming on. I get so afraid of having an attack that . . . although no symptoms actually occur, I start to sweat, get a dry mouth, and have sinus trouble."

Besides these painful sensations, Diane suffers social discomfort from her asthma. She suspects that "people think that I'm making these things up. I have an older sister who says that I brought on every asthma attack in order to avoid responsibilities. That idea really makes me angry." She is acutely sensitive to the social messages that her asthma attacks can convey:

> Yesterday, I went to church, and they had incense burning because of Advent, so I immediately took out my inhaler and put it on the pew. I was feeling really uncomfortable about being there because I hadn't been there for a month, so I figured . . . this would be a good excuse. . . . This became a big thing, like "I'm going to have a hard time breathing, because I'm different from the rest of you." As I was doing that, I knew in a way that I was playing games, but yet that's what I wanted to do.

Diane also suffers from "stomach pains." The first appeared three years ago, when she was laid off from a number of different jobs and spent ten months unemployed. They have gotten worse in the past six months. The stomach pains typically last about one hour, although the accompanying diarrhea may last the entire day. At their worst, Diane reports, the pains are "agonizing, tearing, like my stomach is being pulled apart." But she also describes a more frequent, milder stomach pain as a response to interpersonal conflicts and loneliness: "In my office, there are a lot of fights—who was supposed to do what, whose job it was. . . . After these fights, I'll have trouble with my stomach. It feels like it's in knots. I'll have trouble eating." She describes the first night she spent alone after ten consecutive evenings of church activities:

> I panicked, I felt really odd. . . . I was just trying to do things like clean my room, but I couldn't even do that, because I had this incredible feeling of anxiety . . . I was very tense, my stomach was in knots. It felt like withdrawal symptoms—very bizarre.

Diane's other symptoms don't actually cause pain, but they are bewildering and disruptive, and they communicate messages similar to those conveyed by her asthma and stomach pains. She has found herself at times unable to breathe, speak, or even see. She attributes these episodes to allergies, hyperventilation, or "nerves." As a fifteen-year-old high school sophomore, for example, she remembers waiting for the morning bus, nervously contemplating the play she would later rehearse at school. She noticed that "first, my ears began ringing. Then, my knees gave. I fought it, but my vision became dimmer. I thought I would pass out." She actually could not see for about ten minutes. She recalls a mysterious inability to speak during a church service when she was twenty-four years old: "I was reciting from a memorized text. Then, I just couldn't say it," because she had apparently lost control over her throat muscles. Recently, Diane had to leave work because she found it difficult to breathe. "An incident occurred when a lot of people neglected their filing chores. I was left with their job. But I'm allergic to carbon. . . . I was having trouble breathing, so I left work after that for the day." During the same period, a heavy smoker in her office returned from vacation. While he was gone, she had "had an unusually good week—very few problems breathing. When he came back, these problems reappeared. Whether it was due to smoke in the air, or just his presence, I don't know."

These vivid accounts demonstrate how Diane connects her physical symptoms to problematic relations with her friends and family. In these accounts, her symptoms continually intrude in every sphere of Diane's life. But although her symptoms are annoying, they are not significantly disabling. Although they appear in a wide variety of social situations, the pain or discomfort they cause usually lasts no longer than one or two hours.

Diane's symptoms matter to her not so much because of their brute physical pain, but rather because of their ability to represent her social world. Her pain symptoms convey, in metaphoric though inescapable terms, the frustration she experiences in her relations with friends and family. This occurs in three ways. To begin with, Diane feels condemned by virtually her entire social world for not meeting certain standards of behavior or achievement. She is acutely aware of not conforming to the image of a good daughter, parishioner, or secretary which others hold up as an ideal. She sometimes joins this chorus of condemnation and uses her symptoms to communicate the basic message that something is wrong with her life. That she locates the problem in her body—that is, in herself—instead of in these restrictive social relations, mirrors her harsh self-condemnation.

Diane's world also seems unreceptive to direct protest or attempts to change it. Her symptoms thus persist as one of the few legitimate forms of resistance, since with her symptoms she can escape certain situations or gain the sympathy of co-workers and family members. Therefore, both the marker of troubling relationships and the attempts to change them appear in the internal spaces of the body—usually considered in our culture the ultimately private, nonsocial domain.

Finally, Diane's symptoms play a dramatic role in the stories she tells about her life. She narratizes her experience to demonstrate that resentment and social conflict yield painful bodily symptoms, often within minutes. Her symptoms thus furnish a compelling commentary on her unsatisfying and stifling social relationships. The rest of this case study builds on these stories. It analyzes Diane's symptoms as both a reaction to particular conflicts and a symbol of her general social discomfort—even more, a public symbol conveying that meaning to the people around her.

Family Relations and Pain

"Who do I love the most? The one who is sick, until she gets better; the one who is gone, until she comes home."

—Diane's mother

To specify how Diane reacts to particular social conflicts through a "vocabulary of symptoms" demands a closer examination of her immediate family, the context where her symptoms first appeared. Although she currently lives independently, Diane remains physically close to and very emotionally involved with her family. She lives in the same immediate neighborhood as her aunt's family, while her siblings, parents, and the rest of her relatives live close by. Both her parents are practicing Catholics of Latvian, German, and Irish descent. Both have high school educations. Her father has worked as a truck driver and construction foreman and is currently a night watchman in a local industrial park. Her mother was a receptionist at a real estate office and now works in the data entry division of a local electronics firm. Two of their four children still live at home, Rhonda (age sixteen) and Tim (age eighteen). Diane (age twenty-eight) shares a two-bedroom apartment with another woman, while her older sister Leslie (age thirty-one) is married.

Like most families, the Redens have developed their own characteristic ways of understanding and reacting to physical illness. But unlike many other families, they have an extraordinarily diverse set of chronic symptoms to deal with. Diane's father suffers from chronic (but nondisabling) back and neck pain, sinus headaches, and possibly emphysema. Her mother has complained of a "nervous stomach" since Diane's childhood. She has recurrent urinary tract infections and is clinically hypertensive. She had a ruptured bladder around the time of Diane's birth and was sick for a year. In Diane's words, her mother also has "angina, something wrong with her heart, but she won't go to a cardiologist—she just doesn't want to know. Her father died when he was fifty-four, and now she is fifty-three. He died of heart problems, and she is nervous about that." When she feels these angina pains, Diane's mother "gets very quiet and pale. She just goes away. . . . She doesn't take care of herself, doesn't take her blood-pressure medicine. She has passed out a couple of times at work. . . . She likes to be a martyr."

The Reden children also suffer from various chronic ailments. At different times, Diane, Leslie, and Tim have all experienced painful jaw movements. Leslie has migraine headaches, and during stressful periods they occur as frequently as once every two weeks. Rhonda, the youngest child, was diagnosed with asthma last year and claims she has a "heart murmur," although there have been no positive findings. Diane remembers, however, that when Rhonda was only four years old, she would say, "I'm having chest pains—take me to my special doctor," that is, her pediatrician at a local hospital. Finally, Tim suffers from chronic ichthyosis (dry skin).

Multiple and chronic symptoms have become stabilized in the lives of almost every member of the Reden family. Moreover, illnesses were even accorded a certain esteem in this household. Diane remembers her mother telling her as a child, "Who do I love the most? The one who is sick, until she gets better; the one who is gone, until she comes home." Diane grew up relying on this vocabulary of symptoms to express love, jealousy, closeness, insecurity, and all the other normal family emotions. Her memories of childhood ailments, therefore, focus not so much on actual physical pains as on the painful family relations that accompanied these symptoms.

For example, a stay in the hospital when she was five years old is now told as a story of betrayal and jealousy. Her mother told Diane she was going to have her tonsils taken out, but in fact she had a lump on her neck removed. "I was expecting to stay there overnight, but then I stayed for ten days. It was really horrible. . . . All I remember was crying. My sister was at home, she was getting to watch TV, and I couldn't watch it." During the same year, Diane was diagnosed with pyelonephritis and began a two-year series of weekly clinic visits. She only recently learned from friends that this disease could have been fatal; her mother has never told her this.

Diane's mother became extremely protective because she sensed enormous fragility in her daughter. On the day she graduated from high school, Diane remembers her mother saying, "I never thought you would live this long." Diane's older sister, Leslie, adds, "Diane was a major concern in our mother's life. Diane didn't breathe when she was born, so Mother was always very watchful, expecting the worst." Diane was often uncomfortable and inconsolable as a baby: "Mother always used to say that unless Diane were sick, she couldn't touch or rock her. She just didn't want to be held." Indeed, Diane values the sympathy and protection she has always felt from her mother, but she realizes the danger in it: "My mother tried to make everything perfect, so I was not prepared for life at age eighteen."

Although Diane's symptoms reliably elicited her mother's protection, other family members resented her. "I had one hundred percent of my mother's attention," Diane remembers. "I can't imagine Leslie not wanting more attention. . . . I felt my father resented me, because I spent so much time with Mother." Leslie now admits that she didn't fully understand the meaning of Diane's asthma attacks: "I don't think I took it as seriously as it was. I used to tease Diane when she was wheezing." For her part, Diane felt not only misunderstood but also embarrassed and socially isolated by these attacks. She never wanted to admit that she couldn't keep up with her sisters and their friends or participate in the same kinds of activities.

The physical symptoms Diane experienced as a child and adolescent thus became intertwined with these crucial family relationships. Diane's family is not emotionally demonstrative. "We're not touchy-feely," she says, and Leslie agrees: "People don't talk openly about things, even though they all have insight about it. . . . Everyone usually knows what everybody else is doing, but not what their feelings are." Each child has chosen one other family member with whom to discuss intimate issues. For most of her life, Diane had chosen her mother to play this role, but their "discussions" always took place through the medium of illness. Diane gained security and attention by drawing on a repertoire of physical ailments, and these constituted the vocabulary of symptoms through which they conducted their relationship.

Diane's reasons for maintaining this relationship are clear, but what did her mother gain? One possible answer is hinted at in Leslie's statement that "Mother needed to be needed by Diane" and by their mother's own poignant complaint when Tim graduated from high school, "I'm not a mother anymore, since I have no more children in school." Diane's illnesses intensified her dependence on her mother, and Mrs. Reden felt most assured of her importance to her children when she could comfort them and assuage their pain. During these episodes of sickness, therefore, Diane felt most secure in her mother's love. Looking back on her childhood, Diane herself provides a succinct summary of its lasting effect:

> After being in psychotherapy, I know I associate love and pain. I may have felt that this was the only way I could accept love. Sometimes I'm taken aback by people being nice to me just for the heck of it. . . . Maybe the only way I could feel love was by having some physical need.

Social World and Pain

Diane feels bereft of close friends, and her few social contacts do not give her the support she needs. She does not have a close circle of friends from high school to rely on. Although Diane left home at age twenty-one, she then spent almost a year living at her grandparents' house. Since then, she claims that "almost eighty percent of my life has been at church." She says that before she became active in her church three years ago, she had virtually no adult friends.

Her church provided a ready-made community, but Diane participated in it at a price. She threw herself totally into church activities: for example, one year ago Diane played in a church musical group, helped organize the Christmas concert, and sponsored a woman who was converting to Catholicism. While she remembers being happy at the time, she has begun to reevaluate this period of intense activity. "I was so incredibly busy," she recalls, "and so involved, that when that ended, there was nothing there." Through-out her involvement with the church, in fact, Diane has cycled through periods of busily helping others, feeling accepted, and then feeling used. A period of painful loneliness would predictably follow. In the past few months, Diane has tried to rectify this by dissociating from the church community. When she recently stayed away from church for one month, she was shocked to realize that she had virtually no other source of friendship and close human contact. Moreover, Diane has found that many of her friends from church have made no effort to understand her. One of the few who inquired after her merely told her to stop being so rebellious. Thus, despite belonging to a close-knit community of fellow believers, sharing her interests, class background, and aspirations, Diane continues to feel acutely the lack of an adequate support network. Her church activities have turned out to be an inauthentic way of gaining support.

Her job offers little opportunity for friendships. As a secretary, she is the low-ranking woman in a hierarchical office. Working at an entry-level posi-tion, Diane feels chagrined that people just out of high school soon advance beyond her job level and earn larger salaries. She reports that her boss rigidly controls her work days and often expects her to work overtime on Friday evenings and Saturdays. Diane also resents her boss's sexist attitude. He listens in on her private telephone calls, purportedly to monitor her produc-tivity. He constantly underestimates her work skills, and when she in fact performs competently, tells her, "You're a smart girl, after all." Ever since the only other woman in her office quit, Diane has had no one to commiserate with. Finally, she sees no future advancement in this job. She lists the only things she likes about it: "It's a small office, so I can listen to the radio all day. If we ask, we can be given an extra hour for lunch."

In addition to the objective constraints of job and church, Diane has ex-perienced a number of psychiatric problems that contribute to her social isolation. She currently meets DSM-III criteria for major depressive dis-order, and she also suffers from many of the symptoms of obsessive-compulsive disorder, social phobia, and simple phobia. In the past, she has met criteria for panic disorder, generalized anxiety, and agoraphobia.[2] Her description of particular symptoms underscores her acute interpersonal sen-sitivity. For example, alongside the somatic markers of depression (weight loss of twelve pounds over six weeks, insomnia with early morning waking, loss of energy), Diane suffers from sad and guilty feelings. She pinpoints the source of these feelings: "People are expecting me to be a certain way . . . peo-ple like my family, my friends, my friends from church." According to Diane, they don't understand her depressive mood, which makes her all the more lonely.

She describes the obsessive thoughts characteristic of obsessive-com-pulsive disorder: "I think about people dying, like my family. . . . I feel very guilty about this." In describing her social phobia, she admits that she has always been afraid of situations where others might judge or scrutinize her and that this feeling began when she was fourteen years old. The panic attacks she experienced in the past occurred when things didn't meet Diane's expectations, or when she expected confrontations. She never felt that these attacks came out of the blue. At age twenty-one, she experienced her first episodes of agoraphobia, and they have recurred occasionally since then. The longest episode lasted two weeks. During these episodes, Diane reports that "I can't stand crowds, or other people on buses sitting next to me. . . . I don't like supermarkets and will go out of my way to avoid them." Sometimes even mildly stressful interactions, including "just going to parties," will set off a panic attack. Reflecting more generally on her current state of mind, Diane reports that she has been "extremely distressed" by having her feelings easily hurt, by feeling easily annoyed or irritated, and by feeling that people would take advantage of her if she let them.

This brief list of symptoms and diagnostic categories cannot do justice to the poignant and complex life difficulties Diane now faces. However, one theme does seem to connect her depression, anxiety, and phobias: a pattern of tenuous and unsatisfying social relationships. Whatever the reasons, Diane suffers an acute discomfort with and distrust of other people. In most of her social engagements, therefore, Diane feels caught in a paradox. "The times when I do express myself are really rare," she complains. "I usually adapt to whatever people want me to be . . . I try to change my personality to please the people that I'm with. . . . I've always measured my decisions by what other people thought I should do."

Pain and the Performance of Everyday Life

To please other people, Diane feels she must perform a certain role, meet certain standards, or bend to their will. However, she deeply resents their expectations that she perform for them, and often wishes to sabotage her performance, as if in protest. Performance—within an artificial, alienating, and often subservient role—is the core symbol that unites Diane's physical symptoms to her social world. Viewing her symptoms from this perspective connects the meanings of her pain across childhood and adulthood, and inside and outside her family. The rest of this chapter explores these continuities.

The pressure to perform comes from many quarters. Diane describes the paradox it creates in her family: "My family is the only place where I can be myself, but when I'm there, I always give in to my brother and sister." Her family "performance" consists of playing the role others have chosen for her, such as sick daughter to an overprotective mother. Her church performance was different: "At church, I could present myself as what I wanted to be— dressed nicely, well organized. When I couldn't be that way, that's when I would have symptoms." At church, then, Diane played a self-authorized, perfectionist role, while at home she felt as though she were playing a part in someone else's script. However, her physical symptoms accompany her performance in both cases.

The meaning of her physical symptoms changes according to the type of performance. In the cases above, the symptoms testify to the lack of control Diane experiences in important relations at home and among friends. At other times, however, they take on just the opposite meaning. They also provide a sense of mastery, and Diane traces this meaning of her symptoms to her childhood: "When I was young, the only things that were good were when I was sick. . . . That gave me a tremendous amount of control." Diane still values this as an end in itself, since it counteracts her pervasive feeling that other people and outside events run her life. With the control she gains through illness, Diane feels she can oppose the roles others demand her to play.

In particular, Diane has sometimes capitalized on her physical symptoms in order to influence the audiences who witness her pain to act in a certain way. For example, she remembers becoming sick every Christmas during childhood. Her symptoms, predictably, brought more of her mother's attention to Diane and deflected it from her brother and sisters. She also recalls her grandmother accusing her of playing sick in order to avoid school and her siblings resenting her when she had an asthma attack before her turn to wash dishes or baby-sit.

However, the meaning of her symptoms as an escape from certain performances (a classic example of secondary gain) bears closer examination. Diane freely admits, "To me, I can't distinguish the reality of when I feel sick because I want to escape from when I'm really sick." For example, during a recent rehearsal of her church musical group, Diane began to hyperventilate, in fear of an imminent asthma attack. She left immediately and felt much better, but a few days later she realized she was facing two stressful performances. She was worried about the audience's evaluation of the upcoming concert and also her fellow musicians' evaluation of the program she had designed. Diane thus relied on her symptoms to escape not only an onerous task, but also a literal performance where she felt scrutinized and evaluated.

Diane resents performing on public occasions as well as in the ongoing conventional roles that others require her to play, yet she rarely confronts people with her anger or social discomfort. She instead communicates these reactions through more neutral and disguised media: either her physical symptoms or, intriguingly, objects that are conventionally associated with them. Citing again her return to church after a one-month absence, Diane emphasizes that she did not want to reveal the real reasons for her absence— her dislike of the other parishioners and resentment of their expectations for her. She therefore took out her inhaler and placed it in full view on the back of the adjoining pew. She explains that "I wanted to make it something real medical. That would be a good excuse. I wouldn't have to deal with them or say anything to them." Ascribing her absence to sickness was easier than admitting or explaining her alienation from this community. She thus relied on a tangible symbol of her bodily symptoms—an asthma inhaler—in order to disguise her deeper resentment at the other church members for pressuring her to remain in a restrictive, subservient role.

INTERPRETATION I: PAIN AS PERFORMANCE

Suspicious of the motives of friends; disheartened by her family's restrictive demands; trapped in a dead-end job; intimidated even by her loved ones but angry at them and frustrated by her own acquiescence to their control over her emotional life: the case study must now draw from this complex, contradictory portrait of Diane Reden a few broader lessons for the study of chronic pain. Diane's experience of her physical symptoms displays the use of illness and pain as a medium of communication. The interpretations offered below will illuminate two essential aspects of the "communicative" use of pain: the dialectic between pain and performance and the ways that pain symptoms supply a complex and vital language for social discourse.

Before this theoretical excursus, however, the differences between Diane and other patients with more commonly encountered chronic pain disorders must be restated. Diane's symptoms have rarely caused significant disability or led her to restrict her activities. She certainly faces considerable distress in her life, including family conflicts, anxious or depressed moods, and loneliness and alienation from her friends and co-workers. But in every case, she claims that these life difficulties came first, not vice versa. According to Diane, her pain symptoms did not create her other life problems.

Moreover, Diane's various symptoms do not significantly affect her lifestyle. Despite her pains, she does not avoid any valued activities or hobbies, and she works as quickly, as efficiently, and in the same type of activity as her co-workers. Therefore, her pain does not symbolize a drastic or devastating change in her daily rounds of activities. Having suffered from these symptoms since childhood, she cannot conceive of her pain as the marker of any particular life crisis or transition (unlike, for example, some of the patients profiled by Brody 1987 and Kleinman 1988).

Finally, Diane does not suffer from only one or two overriding pain symptoms. Some patients exploit the metaphorical possibilities of a single physical symptom in order to describe their personality or life dilemmas. For example, a painful, stiff neck becomes emblematic of a tough and unyielding character, or an ulcer symbolizes anger and resentment that one "holds in" and does not express. (For examples of such patients, see Kleinman 1988 and Helman 1985.) With her diverse and changeable symptoms, Diane cannot crystallize her own experience of pain into a single scenario. The meaning of her symptoms therefore cannot arise from such an overdetermined image encompassing both physical sensations and life difficulties.

What sense, then, does Diane make of her symptoms, which neither disable her physically, nor restrict her activities, nor provide a single, tangible symbol for her personal problems? Diane relies on the core symbol of performance to make sense of her symptoms, and in doing so, she illuminates the more general relationship between performance and pain.

Let us first examine how acute pain is performed—a common enough occurrence in most people's lives. This will suggest the special features of chronic pain. The metaphor of performance contains two dimensions: the time frame of the performance and the interactions between audience and performer. Most performances take place over a certain period of "social time." Unlike chronological time, which flows continuously without breaks, social time has a beginning and an end, as well as a varying rate. For example, the drama of a theatrical performance depends on a sped-up presentation of social action, divided conventionally into acts and scenes of varying length, and resolving without remainder at the end of a predetermined period of two or three hours. The very success of a play—judged by its believability or the audience's aesthetic pleasure—arises from this "artificial," socially determined division of time.

Similarly, cases of acute pain inaugurate a highly focused drama, carried along by the structured passage of time. The pain often begins with a trauma or the sudden onset of disease, follows a complex and medically significant course, and eventually ends with restored health, incapacitation, or death. The patient, the patient's family, and health-care providers closely follow these unfolding events. At each stage, they evaluate the severity of the pain, assign it medical or moral meanings, and predict its likely outcomes.

Moreover, the patient who suffers from acute pain is removed from normal time by ceremonial markers such as enforced bed rest and cessation of usual activities. In North American culture, he or she performs a distinct "sick role" with special rights and obligations, such as the right to be excused from normal duties and not be blamed for the sickness and the duty to want to get well and to cooperate with health-care practitioners. But when the episode of sickness ends, the performance (along with its special role) also ends, and the patient returns to presickness roles and resumes the rhythms of normal social time.

The "performer," in the case of acute pain, is the pain itself, while the patient (and others) constitute the audience witnessing the "plot development" of the pain and anticipating its denouement. Because the sick role is temporary, no one expects the patient's enduring behavior patterns or self-image to crystallize around the pain symptoms. The sick role encourages patients to distance themselves from the pain by freeing them of responsibility for the sickness and requiring them to seek out therapies and adhere to a treatment plan.

However, the performance of chronic pain (and chronic illness generally) takes a different shape. The actual symptoms of chronic pain do not lend themselves to the same dramatic conventions. Because the usual markers of severe pain are lacking, people with chronic pain must actively say and do things before specific audiences to reveal their suffering. This leads to a different performative analogy for chronic pain than for acute pain. In this case, the performer is the chronic pain sufferer, and the audience includes his or her family, co-workers, and friends. To extend the metaphor, this audience attends a cycle of performances: the performer is seen again and again by the same audience, acting out the same set of roles. (That performer is interpreted differently, however, by individual members of the audience.) The dramatic interest of these performances of chronic pain, therefore, comes not from new "twists of plot," such as a sudden recovery or relapse, but rather from the gradual revelation of character and motivation and the dynamics between performer and audience.

Thanks to the specific requirements of the sick role, as well as its routine application in our culture, the sufferer of acute pain can reasonably expect to cease being a patient sooner or later. For the chronic pain patient, however, there is no return. Pain itself threatens to become a full-time occupation, and it requires a longer-lasting and more demanding cultural performance. Indeed, chronic pain may eventually stop being a performance separated from the "normal" flow of social life. Whereas acute pain can be analogized to an evening's theatrical performance, chronic pain seems more like a pilgrimage (Frankenberg 1986). Relief from pain becomes an overarching and lifelong goal for such individuals. The search for relief can last for years and include consultations with many different healers. Commanding a large part of the sufferer's emotional and financial resources, involving great hopes and much sacrifice, chronic pain may become the most salient performance of a person's life.

This dialectic between pain and performance becomes clearer in light of an important distinction between the course and the trajectory of an illness. Whereas the *course* of a sickness is defined as its physiological unfolding, its *trajectory* is its social unfolding: the cumulative sum of the patient's performances and performer/audience interactions (Strauss et al. 1985). The notion of a sickness trajectory presents an instructive contrast between the performative dimensions of acute and chronic pain. For acute pain, the trajectory seems naturally appropriate to the course. That is, the changes in role performance, described above as part of the sick role, seem logically called for by the physiological changes produced by the sickness.

This is not the case in chronic pain. The trajectory for a chronic pain patient is inherently problematic, as the details of Diane's life suggest. Certain audiences advance an interpretation of pain-related disability that is different from the one the performer intended. (This happened, for example, when Diane's sister considered her asthma simply as an attempt to avoid family chores.) Indeed, many observable performances, such as verbal complaints, extensive medication, or multiple medical consultations may even be opposed by audiences at home, in the clinic, or in the workplace.

In this chapter the term *performance* has encompassed several different features of chronic pain. While some of these refer specifically to Diane Reden's experience, others shape the lives of most individuals with pain disorders. The following sections review the various ways *performance* has been used in this chapter, and thus clarify what is meant (and what is *not* meant) by the performative aspects of chronic pain.

Performance and the Presentation of Self

The notion of performance refers, first of all, to the dramatic presentation of self in everyday life. Much of our personal identity arises from the reactions of the people around us. All of us, not only those with chronic pain, attempt to guide the impressions we make on others. By controlling the information they have about us, we try to sustain a certain performance—play a desired role—before a given audience (cf. Goffman 1959, 1963).

For people in pain, however, this sort of "impression management" is an especially crucial activity. Chronic pain is a private disorder. Even when it begins with a traumatic accident or major illness, it continues long after these events have faded from people's memory. There are usually few visual emblems—a bruise, cast, or bandage, for example—to announce the presence of pain. The markers of chronic pain are often no more than the words people choose to refer to bodily suffering. People must constantly decide which expressions to use, and who to address, to reveal their pain.

The private, immediate sensation of physical pain thus becomes the occasion for a public "performance." Describing this in dramaturgic terms simply implies that pain sufferers are made extremely aware of the arts of self-presentation. To enact a certain "role" before several "audiences" and to decide what of oneself to place "onstage" and what to keep hidden necessarily become prime concerns for people with chronic pain. However, dramaturgic expressions, such as the "time frame of the performance" or the "social drama" it unfolds, should *not* imply that chronic pain itself is a performance, something voluntarily produced and under one's control. The bodily sensations are not an artifice; instead, people experience pain as an "it," having a powerful reality of its own completely outside their control. Nonetheless, most people with severe and prolonged pain are very aware of the performative dimensions discussed in this chapter: when to hide the pain and when to introduce it into social action. The very ability to do so adds enormous complications to the lives of all in pain. The "social performance" this chapter explores is thus not the pain, but rather people's communications about it.

Pain as Performative Speech

The notion of performance also derives from several contemporary linguistic theories. By talking about painful symptoms and by deciding to reveal them to certain audiences, the person does more than report something about her or his body. The person can actually bring about a change in a given social relationship. Psychologists usually study this under the rubric of "secondary gains," but this term refers more to the practical benefit accruing to the person in pain, rather than the actual rhetorical process through which pain complaints can alter the balance of power or redefine the complex dynamics of a family or workplace.[3]

Of course, the words or gestures that point to physical pain do not always transform the local social world. But regardless of its success, the rhetoric of chronic pain often takes on a certain performative quality. It resembles the type of communication found in a promise or a wedding vow. This use of language does not describe something at a distance; it enacts—or performs—a new state of affairs between the speaker and her audience. Thus the stories Diane Reden tells illustrate a number of both successful and failed "performances" in which she relied on her various pain symptoms to open options for herself within restrictive work and family relations.[4]

Performance and Family Discourse

The metaphors used to describe pain reflect widespread conventions about the body and emotions which are shared by others in the same family or community. Moreover, the reliance on certain metaphors to represent the body can affect the actual experience of physical pain (cf. Scarry 1985). In this sense, chronic pain resembles a more extended performance: a performance *of* cultural and familial idioms, rather than *for* a certain personal goal. Indeed, there is much evidence that family styles can influence the existence or shape of a patient's chronic pain symptoms. For instance, chronic pain patients often have witnessed similar suffering among their kin. In one study, 68 percent of such patients had at least one other family member with chronic pain, compared with 44 percent of patients who were chronically ill but without specific pain complaints. (Violon and Giurgea 1984). In another study, the patient's family, spouse, and spouse's family had significantly more pain complaints than those of matched patients without pain. Intriguingly, even the bodily location of pain was more similar between chronic pain patients and their kin than between non-pain patients and their families (Mohamed et al. 1978).

This research suggests that a "vocabulary of symptoms" may become generalized in a family through the psychological processes of identification and modeling. Hughes and Zimin (1978) specifically showed how such a family-based idiom of distress can influence the pain complaints of children with abdominal pain. These families habitually dealt with conflict and emotional disturbances through bodily sensations, physical explanations, and medico-surgical procedures. The children's chronic pain thus resembled a particular "performance" of the general way their families sanctioned the expression of social conflict.

Let us now return to Diane Reden and the position she occupies within her family. Diane is not the only "identified patient"; for example, several siblings also suffer from physical symptoms, and Diane's mother has recently begun to faint because of her unwillingness to take antihypertensive medication. Diane and Leslie now interpret their mother's behavior as yet another instance of the "vocabulary of symptoms" through which intimate communication takes place in their family. Just as Mrs. Reden most comfortably expresses her love for her children when they are sick, her daughters now think she is relying on these alarming symptoms as the only sanctioned idiom to request love in return.

To deny or to elaborate medical symptoms thus conveys powerful messages about emotional closeness in this family. Diane interprets her mother's symptoms in this light, and she admits that her own pains have been the most reliable way to feel secure in her mother's affection. Diane's illnesses therefore represent the replication and continuation of a particular style of communication: indirect, often unacknowledged, and repetitive. Diane has only elaborated and grown more dependent on this style than the rest of her family. She delivers the most adroit "performances" of her family's general way of communicating.

INTERPRETATION II: THE LANGUAGE OF PAIN

The relationship between pain and performance invites us to rethink how symptoms function as a language. In the stories Diane told about her headaches, stomach pains, asthma, and so on, her symptoms conveyed messages that maintained and even strengthened particular relationships. The meaning of Diane's chronic pain, therefore, lies not only in its biological causes or physiological effects, although these remain crucial for medical treatment. The meaning of her pain lies also in what she is saying through her illnesses and symptoms. Could this meaning also be expressed in words? To whom is it addressed?

Such questions have often occurred to those suffering from (and treating) physical disorders with vague, changeable symptoms that seem to implicate social relationships. In particular, the psychiatric discourse on hysteria—an ancient, almost abandoned term that once might have been applied to Diane's problems—reveals some of the most popular ways of understanding the linguistic characteristics of chronic pain. However, the details of Diane's life also point out the limitations of this received notion (the following discussion is indebted to Forrester 1980).

Contemporary psychiatric nomenclature considers hysteria an anachronistic term for two discrete disorders with both physical and emotional symp-toms: somatization disorder and conversion disorder (a third category, his-trionic personality disorder, does not involve any physical disturbance) (APA 1980). The diagnosis of somatization disorder depends on recurrent and multiple somatic complaints, beginning in adolescence or young adult-hood, and expressed over several years. These complaints often are presented in a dramatic or vague fashion, involving a variety of bodily symptoms, and they are not adequately explained by physical illness or injury. Conversion disorder also features physical dysfunctions not explicable by existing pathol-ogy, but the symptoms are primarily neurological (e.g., paralysis, seizures, blindness), often acute, and clearly the result of the psychological mecha-nisms of primary and secondary gain.

In fact, Diane does not meet the specific diagnostic criteria for either of these disorders. She has just under the requisite number of symptoms for somatization disorder, and her conversion episodes are too few to constitute an enduring pattern. However, the patterns of her pain do resonate with some more general insights about hysteria offered almost one hundred years ago. The nineteenth-century notion of hysteria helps us understand Diane's reliance on a vocabulary of symptoms in her relations with friends and family.

Diane's account of her illness demonstrates that physical symptoms often function as the expression of words in the body, and this viewpoint was a cornerstone of early theories of the origin and treatment of hysteria. Freud wrote that his famous patient Anna O. constructed her own cure out of lan-guage, since "each individual hysterical symptom immediately and per-manently disappeared when . . . the patient had described the [original pro-voking] event in the greatest possible detail and had put the affect into words." Hysteria arises, according to this view, when the memory of a psychic trauma and its strong accompanying affect cannot be expressed in words; when the words are "forgotten," or repressed, and expressed instead as symptoms. However, these symptoms communicate just as effectively as words do, especially in important social interactions, such as between a doc-tor and patient or within a family. The details of Diane's life reveal many instances when symptoms act as the embodied expression of such "lost" words and feelings.

According to the Freudian account of hysteria, symptoms are structured like a language, and they become comprehensible only when decoded (see Gallop 1985). But in this view, the language of the symptom is essentially different from ordinary spoken language. First, the message has supposedly become concealed and distorted. While it definitely conveys meaning, that meaning remains virtually inaccessible by the "hysteric" patient and often unacknowledged by the audience to whom he or she addresses the symptom. Second, the language of the symptom is rigid and repetitive. The hysterical symptom is a piece of language cut off from its original context: a monotonously insistent message repeated before all audiences. This notion of hysteria thus holds that as a patient's words (for troubling memories or feelings) get caught up in the body, they become lost to spoken discourse. As long as the message is conveyed by a symptom, it remains unspeakable and unknowable.

The earliest treatments for hysteria underscore this last point most strongly. Therapy began by retranslating symptoms into words. The patient translated the symptom back into a verbal phrase (of which it had been the recurrent expression), and then placed those words in their proper biographical context. As the patient consciously remembered certain traumatic events, and consciously put into words the accompanying affect, the hysterical symptom (so the theory claimed) would drop away. Thus, for the early Freudians, what takes up a place in the body is lacking from the discourse of the patient, and as it appears in actual speech, it exits the body.

The case of Diane Reden challenges the notion that the embodied message and the verbalized message are mutually exclusive. While certainly relying on her vocabulary of symptoms, Diane also expresses the same messages in ordinary speech. She does not exhibit the ignorance about her symptoms (and the messages they convey) that seemed characteristic of nineteenth-century hysterics.[5] Diane's symptoms do not replace gaps in discourse, since she retains her ability to put into words the same messages her symptoms express. Her verbal messages, however, lack the clarity, authenticity, and power of her bodily messages.

Diane's somatic idiom has thus become stabilized alongside a psychological idiom. This suggests two final implications of Diane's suffering for the study of chronic pain. First, it may initially seem foolish to apply the psychoanalytic model of hysteria to a contemporary case of chronic pain. After all, the florid, dramatic conversion symptoms studied by Freud and his contemporaries have become quite rare among most Western populations. However, chronic symptoms of all kinds—but especially pain symptoms unaccounted for by known pathology—remain an important avenue of communication. They continue to communicate powerful affects and crucial messages about the patient's social life. Moreover, individuals can exhibit such symptoms while remaining psychologically aware of the messages they convey and capable of expressing them in words.

Second, the pain sufferer conveys these messages to particular audiences. That is, the meaning of the symptom (e.g., as threat, incapacitation, marker of old age or lost opportunities) does not stand alone. Instead, it accompanies a message addressed to the patient's most significant friends and loved ones. As the case of Diane Reden points out, these messages are much more complex than the simple search for secondary gains. Each symptom conveys many different messages at once, and these messages (along with the symptoms) may change over the years.

The case study must therefore end on an ambiguous note, since as Diane's life continues, so her symptoms will continue to communicate different and competing themes. They will express acquiescence and resistance to her constrictive roles, resentment, and disguise of that resentment. Any final summary of the meaning of her symptoms is premature. It is even premature to say whether the same dynamic between symptoms and social performances will last, since Diane may someday adopt another idiom (besides the physical symptom) to understand, to change, and to live within her social world. This case study has attempted only to understand her pain symptoms as messages addressed to that world and to demonstrate the importance for anthropological study of chronic pain of considering it as a language in the changing social relationships of the pain sufferer.

ACKNOWLEDGMENTS

I would like to thank "Diane Reden" and her family for speaking to me about their lives with frankness and patience. I am also greatly indebted to Prof. Byron Good, Dr. Arthur Kleinman, Prof. Mary-Jo Good, Dr. Laurence Kirmayer, and an anonymous reviewer for their insightful comments on previous drafts. Portions of this case study were presented at the 1989 Annual Meetings of the Northeastern Anthropological Association in Montreal, Quebec.

NOTES

1. "Diane Reden" is a pseudonym. The names of other family members and certain identifying details have also been changed.

2. These diagnoses are derived from structured interviews using the SADS-L (Schedule for Affective Disorders and Schizophrenia—Lifetime Version). Interviews were held in the author's office. Diane has never been admitted to a psychiatric hospital, although she is currently receiving once-weekly out-patient psychotherapy.

3. Classically, the "gains" of an illness refer to factors other than observable physical findings that contribute to a patient's disability or discomfort. Primary gain refers to the psychological process of avoiding unacceptable affects or reducing anxiety by remaining ill. Secondary gain refers to the obvious interpersonal advantages supplied by symptoms (Freedman et al. 1975). Primary gain usually results from unconscious forces, while the secondary gain is a contingent reward for the pain symptom, which then becomes stabilized through operant conditioning. Because both these theories downplay the importance of the patient's own volition, most case reports of chronic pain patients do not clarify whether the pain sufferer deliberately seeks out these gains (e.g., Bokan et al. 1981).

4. The terminology adopted here comes from Austin (1975). A more precise account of the resemblance between chronic pain and various categories of "performative utterances" is beyond the scope of this chapter. At the least, one must emphasize that chronic pain takes on properties of a "speech act" only after it has

become an acknowledged topic in people's discourse. Moreover, to apply Austin's categories, chronic pain actually performs a "perlocutionary" rather than an "illocutionary" act. That is, it brings about a certain social consequence, but one which is not explicitly contained within the message itself. However, these are not mutually exclusive categories, as Tambiah notes (1985:79).

5. Kahane cogently summarizes Freud's view of the "missing meanings" in the hysteric's bodily symptoms:

> Since hysterics suffered from gaps in their memories, holes in their stories—the sign of repression—Freud's aim was to fill those gaps. Listening closely to the patient's communications—words, gestures, tone—Freud suggested meanings of which the patient was unaware, meanings which, extended to the symptoms, made of them signifiers—i.e., coded representations, that, when understood, formed part of a coherent narrative (1985:21).

REFERENCES CITED

American Psychiatric Association (APA)
  1980   *Diagnostic and statistical manual of mental disorders*, 3d ed. Washington, D.C.: APA.
Austin, J. L.
  1975   *How to do things with words*. Cambridge, Mass.: Harvard University Press.
Bokan, John, Richard Ries, and Wayne Katon
  1981   Tertiary gain and chronic pain. *Pain* 10:331–335.
Brody, Howard
  1987   *Stories of sickness*. New Haven, Conn.: Yale University Press.
Fordyce, W. E.
  1976   *Behavioral methods for chronic pain and illness*. St. Louis, Mo.: Mosby Press.
Forrester, J.
  1980   *Language and the origins of psychoanalysis*. London: Macmillan Press.
Frankenberg, R.
  1986   Sickness as cultural performance: Drama, trajectory, and the pilgrimage root metaphors and the making social of disease. *International Journal of Health Services* 16(4): 603–626.
Freedman, Alfred, Harold Kaplan, and Benjamin Sadock
  1975   *Comprehensive textbook of psychiatry–II*. Baltimore: Williams and Wilkins Co.
Gallop, Jane
  1985   Keys to Dora. In *In Dora's case: Freud—hysteria—feminism*, Charles Bernheimer and Claire Kahane, eds., 200–220. New York: Columbia University Press.
Goffman, E.
  1959   *The presentation of self in everyday life*. Garden City, N.Y.: Doubleday Anchor Books.
  1963   *Stigma: Notes on the management of spoiled identity*. Englewood Cliffs, N.J.: Prentice-Hall.

Good, B.
1977   The heart of what's the matter: The semantics of illness in Iran. *Culture, Medicine and Psychiatry* 1:25–58.
Helman, C.
1985   Psyche, soma, and society: The social construction of psychosomatic disorders. *Culture, Medicine and Psychiatry* 9:1–26.
Holzman, A. D., and D. C. Turk, eds.
1986   *Pain management: A handbook of psychological treatment approaches.* Elmsford, N.Y.: Pergamon Press.
Hughes, M. C., and R. Zimin
1978   Children with psychogenic abdominal pain and their families. *Clinical Pediatrics* 17:569–573.
Kahane, Claire
1985   Introduction (part two). In *In Dora's case: Freud—hysteria—feminism*, Charles Bernheimer and Claire Kahane, eds., 19–32. New York: Columbia University Press.
Kleinman, A.
1986   *Social origins of distress and disease: Depression, neurasthenia, and pain in modern China.* New Haven, Conn.: Yale University Press.
1988   *The illness narratives: Suffering, healing, and the human condition.* New York: Basic Books.
Kotarba, J.
1983   *Chronic pain: Its social dimensions.* Beverly Hills, Calif.: Sage Publications.
Menges, L. J.
1981   Psychological aspects of chronic pain. In *Persistent pain: Modern methods of treatment* (vol. 3), S. Lipton and J. Miles, eds., 87–88. New York: Grune and Stratton.
Minuchin, S., B. Rosman, and L. Baker
1978   *Psychosomatic families: Anorexia nervosa in context.* Cambridge, Mass.: Harvard University Press.
Mohamed, S., G. Weisz, and E. Waring
1978   The relationship of chronic pain to depression, marital adjustment, and family dynamics. *Pain* 5:285–292.
Scarry, E.
1985   *The body in pain: The making and unmaking of the world.* New York: Oxford University Press.
Strauss, A., et al.
1985   *Social organization of medical work.* Chicago: University of Chicago Press.
Tambiah, S. J.
1985   *Culture, thought, and social action: An anthropological perspective.* Cambridge, Mass.: Harvard University Press.
Turk, D. C., et al.
1983   *Pain and behavioral medicine: A cognitive–behavioral perspective.* New York: Guilford Press.
Violon, A., and E. Giurgea
1984   Familial models for chronic pain. *Pain* 18:199–203.

CHAPTER FIVE

Chronic Illness and the Construction of Narratives

Linda C. Garro

I'm hoping to write a book or something about my experiences. That's why I kept all these records and notes. I just hope my history gets out there to help someone else. No one should have to live in this turmoil and be told there is nothing wrong with them.

So in terms of how TMJ has affected my life—radically, totally, entirely. I'm not sorry about all the parts of it, but there are parts I regret, and I'm especially angry at the medical establishment for taking away what worked for me, for making me think I was psychologically impaired.... These must be awful stories. These are stories of medical abuse.

The above statements were made by two women whose illness narratives are the focus of this chapter. These two narratives come out of a series of interviews held with people suffering chronic pain and/or dysfunction that they linked, to varying extents, to the temporomandibular joint (TMJ) in the jaw. The participants were members of a support group. While most referred to their problem simply as TMJ, some referred to other difficulties in addition to TMJ. For example, in the two narratives presented here, one identified her primary problem as a "cranial injury" that led to problems with the TMJ, and the other used the label of TMJ.

People diagnosed with a TMJ problem typically report pain in the jaw joint area, although other symptoms may be attributed to TMJ as well (see Fricton et al. 1985). As a condition requiring treatment, TMJ is most actively claimed by the profession of dentistry (Griffiths 1983), and specialization by dentists in the treatment of TMJ is growing. Overall, perhaps the most striking feature of TMJ is the lack of consensus on just about any aspect of the disorder (Moss, Garrett, and Chiodo 1982; Von Korff et al. 1988b). There is little agreement in the professional literature on etiology, pathophysiology, and treatment (De Boever 1979; Griffiths 1983). There is no formal certification for practitioners providing TMJ care. The term *TMJ specialist* is used in this paper to refer to a health professional who claims the ability to treat TMJ. Many of the individuals interviewed recounted a long, complex history, both prior to receiving a diagnosis of TMJ and after diagnosis, of searching for effective treatment.

Thirty-two participated; all but five were women. This reflects the composition of the two support groups, and also the finding that many more women than men seek specialized treatment for TMJ (Franks 1964; Marbach and Lipton 1978). As the individuals interviewed were all support group members with long term problems associated with TMJ (one year or longer in duration), this sample is not representative of the population of all individuals with TMJ-related pain and/or dysfunction. The types of experience described here are likely more representative of the minority of patients who develop chronic TMJ problems, which has been estimated to include up to 15 percent of patients (National Institute for Dental Research 1990:112).

Both semistructured, open-ended interviews and fixed-response pain and symptom questionnaires were used. During the first part of the interview, people were asked to talk about their experiences with TMJ and chronic pain. They usually responded by telling the story of their illness—how it started, its course, and the search for diagnosis and cure. They described how these events and the effects of TMJ became integrated into their ongoing lives. Thus, these stories are more than illness histories, more than the recounting of events. They are not stories in the conventional sense of being told all at once and in a fixed sequence, but they are stories in that they are inseparable from the ongoing stories of people's lives (see Brody 1987; Murphy 1987; Sacks 1985). What emerged from an interview was not simply the story of an illness, but the story of a life altered by illness.

As people talk during the interview about their experiences, past events are reconstructed in a manner congruent with current understandings; the present is explained with reference to the reconstructed past, and both are used to generate expectations about the future (see Williams 1984; Kelley 1986). This process of reconstructing the past and constructing the present and future occurs throughout the whole interview. In this chapter, the interview material is organized and presented in a way that allows for comparisons across the two narratives as well as identifying similar themes across the set of all narratives. Similarities are present in the types and sequencing of events that people describe as making up their illness histories and in the ways people talk about the impact of chronic pain on their lives.

The two narratives presented illustrate these commonalities. Yet they also defy comparison, offering unique accounts of lives profoundly changed as a result of their experiences with chronic pain and TMJ. Underlying the approach taken here is a tension between representing the complex and particular nature of the individual narratives while identifying similarities in structure and themes across narratives.

RECONSTRUCTING ILLNESS HISTORIES

Similarities across the narratives reflect the process of seeking care for an ill-defined, hard-to-diagnose, and difficult-to-treat condition, such as TMJ, in the context of the American health-care system. As pointed out earlier, most participants recounted a long, often complex, history leading up to the diagnosis of TMJ. For problems now seen as linked to TMJ, individuals often reported being given alternative diagnoses or explanations, including that their pain had no organic basis and was of psychological origin. A striking feature across a number of these stories is perseverance in seeking treatment and relief from pain.

The way in which individuals reconstructed their illness histories followed a pattern that can be depicted as a series of stages. The stories typically start by establishing the genesis of the illness (Williams 1984:180) within the context of a particular explanatory model (Kleinman 1980). A single precipitating event or factor was usually identified, although frequently the contributions of other factors were also detailed.

The next stage covers the period between the genesis to the realization that the physical symptoms are a major disruption in the person's life. In the interviews, this period was described as being as short as a few days or weeks or as long as many years, even dating from birth in a couple of cases. Often, intervening events were seen to affect the course of the illness. The end of this stage marks a major transition. Prior to the realization that their illness represents a serious life disruption, individuals may or may not have sought treatment. Regardless, after this realization, the search for treatment assumes a different quality. Before, the pain and/or dysfunction were often in the background. After, the search for diagnosis and relief from pain comes to the fore.

The stage following realization is characterized by the search for diagnosis and ends with the acceptance of the TMJ diagnosis by individuals. Much variation exists for the number of health professionals seen, with slightly over half consulting four or fewer practitioners prior to receiving a diagnosis of TMJ. However, others saw a number of different practitioners and were often given alternative diagnoses or told that there was no organic problem. This search-for-diagnosis stage was often described as a series of ups and downs until the problem was identified as TMJ and accepted as such by the person. This stage may or may not end when a practitioner gives a diagnosis of TMJ. Some did not accept the diagnosis of TMJ as their primary problem at the time of initial diagnosis, or they vacillated between accepting the TMJ diagnosis and exploring other possibilities. At times this vacillation continued even while they were being treated for TMJ. During the interview, a few expressed uncertainty that TMJ was their key problem. Yet many reported feeling relieved upon receiving a diagnosis of TMJ because that meant there was a physically based and potentially treatable illness (see Berger and Mohr 1967:68). This feeling of relief was sometimes followed by disillusionment when there was no improvement in their condition after treatment.

The last stage is the search for effective treatment. Costs of care were often reported to be prohibitive. Some stressed that TMJ is typically classified as a dental problem rather than a medical one, and therefore treatment costs are not covered by most medical insurance programs. Even so, most persisted in seeking effective treatment, at times consulting a variety of practitioners espousing quite different theories and treatments for TMJ and chronic pain. Seeking relief, they often went outside the professional treatment system to alternative health practitioners. At the time of the interview, some were still actively trying out alternatives, others were not sure where else to turn for relief, and still others reported beneficial effects from their current treatment and an intention to continue with it.

The majority were receiving care from dentists and/or practitioners specializing in physical manipulation techniques (chiropractors, physical therapists, massage therapists, osteopaths, and myotherapists). Within the thirty days preceding the interview, fifteen (47 percent) reported consulting both a dentist and practitioner specializing in physical manipulation techniques, five (16 percent) reported visiting only the former, and eight (25 percent) only the latter. Mouth splints or appliances were the most common form of treatment provided by dentists, although more extensive dental or orthodontic work was reported by some.

When asked how the past six months compared to the worst they had felt with TMJ, fourteen (44 percent) stated they felt much better; eleven (34 percent) stated they felt somewhat better; and six (19 percent) said that the past six months were equal to the worst. One person said her problems occurred so cyclically that it was not possible to make a judgment.

Although some expressed optimism when asked about future management of TMJ and pain, no one foresaw a life free of the effects of TMJ. For those in chronic pain, the story is a continuing one. New events and information are either incorporated in the current construction or provide the impetus for revising the narrative to accommodate new interpretations.

THE ONTOLOGICAL ASSAULT OF CHRONIC ILLNESS

In addition to shared experiences in the seeking of care, individuals commonly faced similar challenges through the significant disruption and alteration in their lives caused by chronic illness and pain. A number of studies have documented the disruption caused by an inability to carry out social roles within the family and the workplace (Williams 1987) and the strategies used to maintain the appearance of normality or to adjust to diminished capacity (Wiener 1975; Reif 1973; Strauss and Glaser 1975). More fundamentally, the disruption of the taken-for-granted world of everyday life (Berger and Luckman 1966; Quinn and Holland 1988) caused by chronic illness can be seen as "nothing less than an ontological assault" (Pellegrino 1979:44), affecting the concept of self and not merely the performance of activities.

Through their stories, people conveyed how the lived experience of chronic pain and dysfunction affected the way they thought about themselves, their lives, and their future. Goals, plans, and expectations about life were often radically revised in the face of an illness with no foreseeable end. As people tell their narratives, not only is the past reconstructed to account for illness, but the view of the present and future is also evaluated and constructed anew. These narrative projections into the future, the person's life plan (Brody 1987) or life sketch (Nardi 1983), reflect the perceived constraints of chronic illness. The life plan as changed by illness can be contrasted with the life plan held prior to illness, giving a before-after quality to the narratives. Nevertheless, to see chronic illness solely in terms of loss is too simple; almost always there is a reaction to preserve one's identity (Sacks 1985:4). Much of what people told us concerned their attempts to maintain a sense of self and purpose in the face of this profound life disruption (see Brody 1987; Bury 1982; Kelley 1986:665; Kleinman 1986, 1988; Sacks 1985; Williams 1984:179). Indeed, this "dual nature of sickness—the way it can make us different persons while we remain the same person" (Brody 1987:x) is an integral part of the narratives told by sufferers of chronic illness.

Questions about the authenticity of the pain experience, especially when raised by medical professionals, represent yet another ontological challenge to the integrity of the self. Attributing the pain to a malfunction of the mind rather than of the body implies that it is the sufferer who is to blame for both the pain and for the failure of the practitioner to achieve a cure (Eisenberg 1981:245; Fabrega and Manning 1972; Kotarba and Seidel 1984). In response to these attributions, informants often made statements such as the following and those appearing at the head of this chapter:

> And there are so many insidious factors . . . like the reaction from the medical establishment. It's like you're somehow doing this to yourself, so in addition to your pain, you've got someone telling you you're crazy. . . . It's like it's your fault. You obviously have some character defect because you can't handle your stress like everyone else. Stress is not the problem here . . . being thrown through a car is the problem.

The "ontological assault" caused by chronic illness also challenges other aspects of the relationship between self and body. Because of illness, the body becomes a problem, no longer "the subject of unconscious assumption, but the object of conscious thought" (Murphy 1987:12). Illness transforms the "lived body," in which self and body are unified and act as one in the world, to the "object body," where the body is a source of constraint and is in opposition to self (Gadow 1980). People respond to the restraints and demands of the body in different ways, and this is reflected in their narratives.

The themes discussed in this section are not the only examples of shared content across the illness narratives, but they are among the most salient.[1] Along with the narrative structure outlined in the previous section, they provide the analytic framework for discussing the two narratives. Each reconstructed illness history is followed by a discussion of the response of each person to chronic illness and pain. The life plans of both have been radically altered as a result of their experiences; both have been confronted with the view that their problems are psychogenic; both have developed a new relationship with their bodies.

The two narratives presented here are quite complex, as are others obtained in the study. These two narratives were selected primarily because they represent quite different responses to the "ontological assault" of chronic illness and pain and thus provide an illustration of the degree of comparability and diversity occurring across the interviews. In addition, each gave permission to interview a key treatment provider at the time of the interview. Both health-care practitioners, one a physician and the other a dentist, basically concurred with the interpretation of TMJ given by their patients. This raises a flag of caution to those who would dismiss the interpretations of lay people because they are not based in the "objectivity" of medicine.

The narratives are presented from the perspective of the person interviewed. In each, the contributions of conflicting and complementary explanatory models are evaluated within the context of the current model. Except as expressed by the narrator, there is no weighing of the evidence for or against particular interpretations; rather, the focus is on the process of narrative construction, using the stories told by two individuals, and how they view their "changing relationship to the world and the genesis of illness within it" (Williams 1984:175).

MARY BARTLETT'S STORY

When I first met Mary ("Molly") Bartlett, the only visible sign that something was not quite right was the way she conscientiously maintained her posture throughout the long interview session and the extremely careful movements of her head and body. This session and the one that followed occurred right after visits to her chiropractor, and Molly explained that through attention to body position and movement she was attempting to prolong the benefits of treatment. In marked contrast to her body's lack of spontaneity, Molly laughed, cried, and expressed anger at various times during the course of the interview. Overall, she was cheerful and pleased to participate in the study, stating she hoped that her story might somehow help others faced with similar problems, a hope shared by many of the other participants.

Molly is married with several children. She is currently on long-term disability from her job as an aide in a nursing home. She has been away from work for approximately two years. For the past twenty years, with the exception of one week, not a day has gone by when she was free of pain or other symptoms. Yet, Molly sees herself as having fought a successful battle against pain through her efforts to maintain as normal a life as possible.

The narrative constructed by Molly centers on her understanding of the physical basis of her problems. Molly sees her pain and other symptoms as caused by structural imbalances, localized primarily in the cranium. Molly clearly identifies an initial head injury as the starting point for her problems, with additional trauma and physical stress seen as contributing to further structural imbalance that was expressed through a variety of initially puzzling symptoms. Molly currently receives medical care from an osteopath and a chiropractor, both of whom specialize in cranial manipulation. The stated objective of this treatment is to manipulate the cranial structure, moving it back into the position occupied prior to the original trauma. As this is done, Molly experiences a reversal of symptoms. At the time of the interview, she reported experiencing the same symptoms as felt approximately six years after the initial trauma. Molly often uses the metaphor of a road, describing how as her symptoms worsened she came down the road, while now, as she improves, she is coming back up the same road.

Genesis

Molly now dates the genesis of her difficulties to a bicycle accident that occurred some thirty years ago in her mid-teens. In this accident, she fell, hitting the right side of her head against a curb. She lost consciousness and only remembers waking up in her bed at home later. The right side of her face was bruised and she had very strong headaches for months afterward. Her family doctor, who was consulted several times after the accident, said her headaches were normal, given the type of injury she had sustained. In time, the headaches diminished both in frequency and intensity, and while Molly continued to have them, she explained, "I found . . . as long as I kept active, I didn't have to realize what was happening."

Talking about the importance of this injury for her subsequent physical problems, Molly states:

> You know, no one records a head injury, whether you've fallen off the changing table, whether you've fallen off your bike. No one ever records those things, and those things can lay dormant until later on in life when there is [physical] stress and the muscles just say, I can't do it anymore.

From Genesis to Major Disruption

The ten years following the injury were relatively healthy ones for Molly. Even so, looking back, she now thinks that several incidents and symptoms are linked with the head injury. These include muscle problems with her leg, learning difficulties in school, and episodes when she would cry for no apparent reason. Her doctor and parents attributed the muscle problem to her heavy involvement in sports, and her mother often commented that her other difficulties were just part of the process of growing up. Visits to the dentist also caused problems. Twice, after routine fillings, Molly had to return to the dentist because of pain. She states now that "it was probably the first sign that there was really something drastically . . . not stable within the structure, but I didn't know anything about TMJ."

After graduating from high school, Molly married and had a couple of children by her early twenties. These pregnancies were difficult ones, which Molly now sees as causing further structural imbalance in her body. She had muscle problems in her legs which often affected her ability to walk, but she states that at the time "I just figured that this was something that every woman goes through, so I never made an issue."

Slightly over a year after the birth of her youngest child, Molly went to work part-time at a nursing home to supplement the family income. Two years later she switched to a full-time position. In her job she often helped move people and carried out other physically demanding tasks. Molly sees this as exacerbating the damage caused to her head by the bicycle injury. Indeed, she feels that if she had not worked in a job that placed so much physical stress on her head, neck, and back, her problem would have remained a minor one, with symptoms only of headache and leg, arm, and neck pains, for which she would not have sought medical treatment. Shortly after her twenty-seventh birthday, the level of pain and dysfunction she felt went from minor to major.

One day, while she was working, she reported that suddenly it "felt like someone came and hit me on the right side of the head." Her whole right side was affected, with her arm, leg, and face feeling numb, much "like novocaine wearing off." She was unable to perform normal activities. The staff doctor took some X rays and referred her to a neurologist, who blamed the problems on a pinched nerve and said she would recover completely.

Although she quickly improved, Molly sees this incident as a turning point. She states:

> Once I tipped, once this muscle finally let go, all the TMJ symptoms came into effect. The whole cranial had to shift to accommodate me being tipped to the right . . . the whole muscle tone changes because of being kicked out of alignment. Neurologically, there's a complete change. I had to learn not to do things because I could aggravate those muscles.

The Search for Diagnosis

For Molly what followed after she "tipped" was fourteen years of uncertainty about what was wrong with her. Her history through this period is a complex one of variable symptoms and of seeking treatment from a number of practitioners. At first, she continued to have problems on her right side and repeatedly consulted the same neurologist. Over the three years that she saw him, he prescribed heat treatment and traction. He suggested the possibility of arthritis and at one point recommended surgery "to relieve the pressure around the nerves." A chance comment that her work could be aggravating injury originating in a previous whiplash raised the possibility in her mind for the first time that the bicycle accident could be linked to her present problems. This possibility was not investigated further at this time.

Concerned about the possible dangers associated with surgery, she discontinued her visits to the neurologist. During the time she had seen him, she suffered a variety of other apparently unrelated symptoms of varying duration—difficulty chewing and swallowing, gum problems, bladder control problems, frequent bowel movements, and difficulty pronouncing certain sounds. At the time of the interview, these were all linked to the head injury. She had gum surgery and saw her family physician several times, in particular to check out the bladder and bowel problems. No sign of infection or disease was found. Other than these visits, she consulted with no other practitioners at this time. She explained: "I'm not one to beat down a doctor's door." Her main concerns were the headaches and the continued pain and weakness on the right side of her body. Her other problems at this time were not severe enough to cause alarm. She found herself limited in everyday activities, substituting crocheting and knitting for bowling and badminton and making drastic changes in her housework patterns so she would be able to keep working. She did continue to work and at one point had three years of perfect attendance.

Five years after the incident at work, she was involved in a traffic accident that involved a blow to the chin. At the hospital "they picked up my malocclusion, of the lower jaw being back . . . and at the time I told them that's how I was." At the time, she paid little attention to this piece of information, but later it became supporting evidence for TMJ.

After six weeks of recuperation, she was back at work. Her symptoms worsened. From the vantage of the present, she explains: "I must have been hit back more than I was already back," causing her cranial structure to go even further out of alignment. A difficult pregnancy soon after the accident was seen later as adding further stress on the cranial structure. The eight-year period from after the birth of her last child until she was diagnosed as having TMJ was filled with both numerous symptoms and many visits to physicians. Recalling this period, she made the following two statements:

> My whole system was so sensitive that everything was overworking. It was just that. I had everything going against me. Everything just went. At this time I didn't realize that all my problems were just one problem.

> I was going from one problem to another problem and no one could give me any answers. They did tests. They found nothing wrong with me.

A sampling of the practitioner visits she made during this time, for problems she now sees as being related to TMJ, follows. Unless specifically mentioned, for none of these visits were any significant findings reported. Because of her headaches and right-side numbness, she was referred by her family physician to a neurologist, who did an electroencephalogram (EEG) and computed tomography (CT) scan. She went to the emergency room at the hospital several times because of difficulty breathing due to swelling of her tongue. She had a dilation and curettage to regulate her heavy menstrual flow. She saw her family physician again about her frequent bowel movements. She saw two, perhaps three, otolaryngologists about her tongue, sinus, and upper-respiratory problems. One of them suggested that perhaps the problem was caused by a hormone imbalance and suggested that she take birth-control pills. She saw an ophthalmologist about her watery eyes. She consulted with an orthopedic surgeon, who put her in a back brace and gave her cortisone shots. This surgeon also suggested surgery to reattach a muscle in her right leg, but Molly demurred, saying it couldn't be a detached muscle because the weakness and numbness were not constant. Throughout these visits she presented only selected symptoms to each physician for fear of being labeled a hypochondriac. Describing her feelings at this time, she said: "What I couldn't understand is why I had to give up everything but yet nothing was wrong with me. It was like you wanted to shake them and say, 'Can't you see what's happening to me?'"

The culmination of these feelings occurred after a visit to a pain-management clinic recommended by her co-workers. Molly went through a battery of evaluations over several days, and afterwards, she recounts:

> I had all the tests done. I'd seen all these specialists, just to be told by a woman doctor at the end that I'm a working mother and that I don't know how to handle my life. The day they gave me the outcome of my diagnosis, I got out of the city . . . I pulled the car over and I just started crying. They didn't give me no avenue to go down. It was . . . there's nothing wrong, well, you're out.

Molly refers to the visit to the pain clinic as the "low point" and states that it would have been very easy, then, to give up, go on drugs, or become an alcoholic. Her response was to live just one day at a time and keep busy both at work and at home, "because as long as I keep my mind completely occupied, I don't go into a state of depression or anything."

Her physical problems continued: "And this is how I kept coming down the road, leaving things I knew I couldn't do and not doing them till I got to the point that I couldn't do anything. I couldn't sit. I couldn't stand, and everything was overworking and working wrongly." Her husband suggested that she quit work and try to find out what was wrong with her. Her response was: "Who am I going to see? I'm not going back to the hospital to get rejected." She also felt that she couldn't walk away from an income the family needed "because no one would give me a medical [leave]."

A co-worker recommended that she visit a chiropractor. One of the physicians Molly had seen previously had warned her not to see chiropractors, as she would be left a cripple. "But then I thought, I am crippled. I can't do anything. I'm not living a life, except going to work . . . yet I couldn't share this with anyone. So I said, well, what have I got to lose. That's about the only end of medical I hadn't gone to."

The chiropractor she consulted told her she had classic TMJ with a malocclusion in the jaw that was affecting her entire body. He said he could provide temporary help but that she should see someone to correct the malocclusion. Molly felt that the change after seeing the chiropractor was phenomenal: "I couldn't believe that within two weeks, I had no more headaches, I had no bowel problems." But even better than that: "You don't know what a weight was lifted off my shoulders in the first week of seeing him. This was the first time someone could tell me my problem."

The Search for Effective Treatment

The initial visit to the chiropractor marks the beginning of the final stage of Molly's narrative, the search for effective treatment, which covers the six years preceding the interview. Her chiropractor referred her to a dental clinic where an internal mouth splint was built to help realign the jaw. After starting to wear this, she was much improved. Some weakness on her right side and pains in her leg were the only remaining symptoms. The dentist said that while the headaches had been caused by TMJ, the weakness and pain on the right side were not. After a couple of months, she was told to go without her splint, but whenever she did everything went "haywire" and symptoms returned. The dental clinic did some dental work that involved grinding down some of her teeth. She now feels this led only to further structural imbalance: "they took away that little bit of muscle tone I had that supported me." Molly switched to another dentist, who adjusted the splint, and also started to see a physical therapist.

Although she still had some physical difficulties, Molly felt much improved. Then she broke the mouth appliance, and without it, some of her symptoms flared up. The replacement splint never worked as well as the first. This experience led to the realization that while the mouth appliances were helpful, they were not a solution: "I look at any mouthpiece as a crutch. If that crutch bends, if it wears down, if it breaks, you're back to day one. You've still got your problem."

A son who had been away for several years returned home and was surprised at the extent of his mother's suffering. He arranged for her to see a medical doctor who specialized in homeopathic remedies. The homeopathic physician said he could provide some symptom relief but also referred her to an osteopath who specialized in cranial manipulation.

The osteopath diagnosed serious imbalances in the cranial structure. Molly feels that his treatment was the first time someone dealt with "my main problem, which was the resting position within the head structure."

What causes the different symptoms, Molly says, "was the brain, the nerves giving the wrong information because of where I was resting."

She stopped seeing the chiropractor at this point. Under the direction of the osteopath, the dentist constructed an adjustable mouthpiece to complement the osteopath's treatment. At this point, something remarkable happened. She noticed that she started to repeat symptoms: "I'm reversing the way I came, the symptoms I had, I'm now repeating." Initially frightened by this, she wanted to discontinue treatment, but she was reassured by the homeopathic physician, who told her: "If your body can repeat the symptoms that shows you're going the right way. You stay with it." As treatment continued, she went through all of her symptom history in reverse, finally reaching the point where she was without any problems. In recalling this time, she stated: "It was tremendous. Boy, I never realized that life was so easy going." This experience suddenly ended a week later when "whammo, I wasn't able to walk, I was in a lot of pain and had a high fever."

The interpretation given by the homeopathic physician for these occurrences is that even though the manipulation had succeeded in moving the cranial structure back to the position it held before the bicycling accident, there was so much underlying structural instability that it simply moved out of position again and led to the recurrence of ill health. He thought that over time it should be possible to move her cranium back into its original position and to do it in such a way that her head structure would remain stable. Molly felt that she would be able to tell when the cranial manipulation was appropriate by the symptoms she was feeling. With the exception of the homeopathic physician, it took some time before the others treating her would listen and work within this framework. Molly recognizes that both her problems and their treatment are uncommon and are not taught in medical school. She is grateful to have found practitioners who are willing to listen to her and work to alleviate her suffering.

When the osteopath developed health problems that caused him to cut his practice, he referred Molly to a medical doctor who specializes in osteopathic manipulation. The original osteopath continued to see Molly monthly to monitor her progress. Molly also started to see a chiropractor recommended by the physician. Around this time, approximately a year and a half before the interview, Molly went on short-term medical leave from her job. The physician, the osteopath, and the homeopathic physician all wrote letters stating she was temporarily disabled. With the exception of two brief attempts to return to work, she has remained off work and is now on long-term disability leave. She says that by continuing to work, she was undoing any benefits of the treatment. She explained: "When they manipulate me and get me comfortable, I could do anything, but yet I can't do everything, because if I do something right after they manipulate me, I'm just going to undo what they're helping me to do."

In the six months preceding the interview, the nursing home Molly worked for tried to intervene in her treatment by sending her to an oral surgeon and back to the same pain-management clinic that Molly associates with the low point of her illness history. The oral surgeon noted that there was some malocclusion but said Molly neither had TMJ nor was it responsible for her symptoms. Molly was not surprised by this, as "my problem is a medical problem. It has nothing to do with the teeth." Her visit to the pain clinic resulted in a letter stating that she had a psychiatric condition known as somatization disorder and that there was no organic basis for her problems. After receiving the letter, Molly reported being less upset than she was after the first visit to the clinic, when she did not have an acceptable explanation for what was happening to her. In discussing her experiences with the clinic, Molly places her experiences within the broader context of all TMJ sufferers:

> They call TMJ and head trauma the silent epidemic, and it is. We are mistreated. And this will happen until doctors realize that what happens within the head structure can make things happen throughout the whole body just because that's the information that's coming to it.

Overall, Molly feels she is improving. To use her own phrase, she is coming back down the road. She has gone through the symptoms in reverse for the past two years, and sees herself currently experiencing symptoms that were common during the six-year period immediately after the accident. The asymptomatic periods following a successful cranial manipulation last longer. She describes her current condition: "Right now we are very, very delicately getting there. But there's still no bending because I can wipe out anything within a short minute if I do it." Although she still experiences a lot of pain and dysfunction, she finds it much easier to handle: "Because now I know what my problem is. Before it was frightening in a way . . . because I didn't know why all these things are happening to me and I didn't know how to help myself."

Help-Seeking as Life Plan

It was only after Molly received a diagnosis of TMJ and developed an explanatory model that provided the framework for understanding her physical problems that her life plan changed. Prior to this: "I didn't let into it. I kept going. I never gave in. I wasn't one to stay in bed. I kept doing things even though I didn't feel well." Still, she found this difficult: "The hardest thing is people don't understand what pain I'm in. They say I look so healthy. It's pain day after day after day." She managed by substituting activities she could do for those she could not. Molly identifies herself primarily as a wife and mother; her work is important only as a means of support for her family. Thus, Molly would not leave her job unless she could do so with a medical leave; to do otherwise she saw as irresponsible, given the importance of her income to family finances. She maintained her sense of self by not giving in to the nameless pain, by not allowing it to alter her life plan significantly.

Her current life plan and her view of the future are centered on health seeking. Molly has wholeheartedly accepted the obligations of the Parsonian sick role to try to get well and to seek out competent help and cooperate in efforts to restore health (Parsons 1951). Although her main identity as a wife and mother has not been negatively affected by the revisions to the life plan, many other aspects of her life changed. She did go on leave from her job. Yet this occurred at a time when Molly felt in better health than she had during most of the time she had worked. On the surface this seems contradictory, but Molly explained that her job counteracted the treatment she was receiving, leading to further instability in cranial structure and interfering with the key treatment goal of moving her cranium permanently back to its normal resting place. Thus, to enable her to regain her health, Molly no longer works at her physically demanding job, but spends much of her day participating in recreational activities or "taking it easy." Activities she enjoyed and used as therapy during earlier stages in her illness, such as swimming and bicycling, have now become an important part of her daily routine. She reports enjoying life more and doing more activities as the amount of time spent in pain diminishes. Being off work on a medical leave lends further support to the life-style she has adopted.

She has devoted much of these past two years to treatment, and she usually receives cranial manipulation on each weekday from either the chiropractor or the osteopathic physician. She also consults the homeopathic physician on an as-needed basis for remedies to counteract the symptoms she is currently experiencing. Molly is receiving what she believes to be the best care available for her condition. She has learned some cranial manipulation techniques and is at times able to treat herself. Although all of her disability income is spent on obtaining treatment, Molly feels it is well spent in the continuing effort to restore her health. At the time of the interview, Molly stated that she hopes to be able to return to work soon and predicts that she will have returned to her "normal physiological resting place" in about five months, adding quickly that she thought the same thing five months ago.

The Body in Control
During the interviews, Molly referred many times to the extreme sensitivity and uniqueness of her body. She frequently mentioned her inability to take pain-relief medications, even in small dosages, as they always put her to sleep. This sensitivity of the body is both at the root of her problem and the means for achieving stability. Molly feels that another person with the same initial head injury and subsequent physical stresses would most likely have developed only chronic headaches and not all the diverse and varied symptoms she has experienced. Yet she feels extraordinarily responsive to her

cranial manipulation treatment. Molly states that while most people respond in two weeks, her response is immediate.

But before Molly settled on her current treatment, hers was a body out of control, a truly anarchic body (Turner 1984). Symptoms would come and go inexplicably. Molly's weight also fluctuated widely. The weight fluctuations were not attributed to any changes in eating or exercise patterns, but rather to changes in her cranial stability. Molly gained weight between the incident at work when she "tipped" until soon after the first visit to the pain-management clinic, when there seemed to be no solution to her problem. She reports losing this weight during the period when she was relying on the chiropractor and mouth appliances and felt relatively pain-free and in good health. Her weight shot back up again at the start of the symptom-reversal stage, and she hopes her weight will go back down once her cranium is stabilized. However, Molly says there is nothing she can do to control her weight. Also, according to Molly, the normal relationship of mind directing the body's actions could be severed at any moment. She reported several instances when she was unable to act at will. One case involved a stranger at a restaurant who choked at lunch. Although Molly knew the correct procedure for saving her, she found herself unable to carry it out and had to tell someone else how to do it. Describing her relationship with her body, Molly said: "You would expect it to do something for you and all at once—you didn't think you couldn't do it, so you went and did it. And all at once you found you couldn't do it and you would have to give in to it."

Although Molly describes her body as not responsive to her thoughts or actions, the relationship appears to be one in which the body has the upper hand—the body is able to influence self more than self influences the body. Changes in her emotions and cognition are often attributed to where she is "resting." She described several incidents when she cried without any apparent reason. It is also not uncommon for her to be affected on a cognitive level. She may be unable to remember anything new, no matter how long she studies or how hard she tries. Molly sees these emotional swings and learning difficulties as the same kind of problems she had as a teenager shortly after the initial head trauma. At times, Molly enters into a "negative stage," when she feels her current treatment is getting her nowhere. She gets very angry toward those who are treating her and wants to give up all treatment. Recently, when Molly has experienced the "negative stage," her husband has suggested she go to the chiropractor so he can move her out of it. Molly comments:

> These are very close, the sleep stage, the cry stage, the negative stage—like I'm not going to go on with it. To heck with them and everything. And then right with that is where you think of things that happened so far back in your life. The only way I can look at it is as an index, and all at once these things are popping out of an index and that's where you're at. Not that you want to feel it

or think it or . . . but that's the nerves that are involved and that's the information that you are getting.

Thus, for Molly, not only does her body affect perceived symptoms and bodily processes but also emotions and cognitive processes. Often the body, not the self, is in control.

Prior to starting her current treatment, Molly had no effective way of dealing with her body. With the constant, yet unpredictable, symptom flare-ups, all Molly felt able to do was to resign herself to a different level of functioning. Her current treatment directly affects her body through physical means. Molly describes the cranial manipulation as bringing her out of symptoms. As control over her body has increased through treatment, so does her control over her activities, and indeed, her life.

Mind and Body

Through much of Molly's illness, she did not know why she was having so many different problems. Worse than that, none of the physicians consulted were able to tell her. The initial visit to the pain-management clinic increased her suffering when she was told she had no organic problem whatsoever. Clinicians specializing in pain had failed to validate her pain experience (see Cassel 1982). After this failure, there seemed to be nowhere else to try.

Molly rejected the suggestion of the pain-management clinic and all other similar suggestions that her difficulties were caused by stress and essentially psychological. Locating her difficulties within the mind was a direct threat to Molly's sense of self. After all, her problems were not minor; they entered into every aspect of her life. The legitimation of her problems as physically based was very important to Molly.

Looking back and reinterpreting the past within her current explanatory framework, Molly is able to give two reasons why her problem was not diagnosed until she reached the chiropractor. The first reason is that most physicians are not trained to pick up problems of head structure. They simply "don't realize that symptoms come from nerves. That where you rest, that's what you're going to have." It can't be picked up by an X ray because "there is no deterioration. The muscles were out of alignment. The whole face was out of alignment." Other individuals interviewed in this study often commented on physician lack of knowledge about TMJ.

The second reason has to do with the extreme sensitivity of her body. The diverse symptoms were masking her true problem, and it was difficult even for the people who are currently treating her to understand how so many symptoms can be related to one basic problem. At one time, the chiropractor wanted to stop treating her because he felt her problem was beyond him. She told him that "any doctor would have felt that way . . . what we're doing is unheard of." The uniqueness of her body and her problem is confirmed by her current treatment. Molly reports the osteopath once said:

> I can't take you to the doctor next door and say, "Look at Molly, look at what this is doing." He said because each doctor that comes out of medical school is taught a certain way and that's the way they practice. He said your kind of problem is never heard of, never heard of there. You are so super sensitive you can tell us everything that is going on. We never had this before. He said, even with myself, when you tell me these things and I find these things happening to you, you know, it isn't supposed to be that way.

Although the response of her body is unique, for Molly, the underlying problem is not. Molly sees herself as an extreme example of people in pain caused by cranial and structural imbalances. Indeed, Molly made repeated comments of concern about others who suffer pain but do not know the cause or who may have been misdiagnosed because of limitations of current medical knowledge and practice:

> and you just wonder, how much of the suffering in this world could be helped if people realized what does happen within the whole system. I'm just wondering, how many people are in institutions because they couldn't handle that kind of pain, you know, that there is something happening that's giving out the wrong information to the body. Like I said, we don't get sick or anything, but it is there. We have all the symptoms, but it isn't a symptom that a doctor can pick up on.

GAIL JOHNSTON'S STORY

This narrative represents a different response to TMJ. During our meetings, Gail Johnston, like many of the people interviewed, was careful with her body and its movements, although not to the degree that Molly was. As Gail is petite, the way she held her body reinforced an impression of physical fragility. At the same time, her statements attesting to the need for individuals to take an active role in managing pain and illness, coupled with her determination to improve her health and her life, belied her fragile appearance.

Gail Johnston holds a university appointment in a department of political science. Involved in both teaching and research, Gail also derives some of her income from external consulting activities.

Gail says that having TMJ has affected her life "radically, totally, entirely." This effect is a multidimensional one. On a physical level, TMJ is linked with pain, upper body weakness, and muscular spasticity throughout her body. Of these three, the pain is the worst, and it is most intense in her jaw area. Other badly affected areas include her neck and cranial area. Over time, she has come to feel pain in her right hip joint and right shoulder blade.

The pain is always present, although it waxes and wanes. It is exacerbated by such everyday activities as eating and talking. The upper-body weakness and spasticity developed later than the pain. Because of the upper-body weakness, she is unable to carry things, such as books or groceries, very far. The spasticity means that at times she will be holding something and suddenly, without intending to, she will let go of it. Gail finds she is always bumping into things, knocking things over, and dropping things.

While she often feels restricted in activities and cut off from goals she would like to achieve, her experiences with TMJ have also led her to consciously reevaluate her life plan and make changes in it. While artistic expression was always an important part of her life, communicating her experiences with chronic illness through her art has become central to her revised life plan. That her life goals are different is seen as a positive effect of TMJ and pain. Gail feels that she has grown through her pain.

To a large extent, Gail constructs her narrative around her interactions with "whitecoats," a term she uses to refer to "the medical establishment." Although she attributes her initial problems with TMJ to physical damage and stress to the right jaw, combined with a possible innate predisposition due to the structure of her palate, a large part of her narrative describes how she progressively became worse through treatment interventions. Gail felt that most of the stories we were being told about TMJ were, like hers, "stories of medical abuse." Through treatment, not only Gail's body but her mental capabilities were negatively affected. Indeed, Gail feels strongly that had she remained a "passive object" and not come to take an active role in managing her pain through meditation, she would no longer be alive.

Genesis

Gail began her history by mentioning two possible contributing factors from her childhood, even though she was unsure whether they were causally related to her development of TMJ. First, she noted that her parents have high soft palates like her own and that they were always in poor health and had many dental problems. She now suspects they might have a minor TMJ problem. In support of this hypothesis, she points out that as a child she often suffered from allergies and headaches. Second, she once ran into a glass door at running speed by mistake, injuring her head.

More central to Gail's reconstructed history were several incidents of head trauma occurring approximately twenty-two years before the interview. Gail described these incidents as representing a history of consistent abuse to the right side of her head. The key incident was a car accident during which Gail heard her jaw crack. In addition, around the time of the accident, Gail had been taking judo lessons, in which she was taught to fall on her right side. That same year she was also accidentally hit on the right side of her head during a judo class.

From Genesis to Major Disruption

After these injuries, even though her headaches worsened, she still saw them primarily as a continuation of childhood health problems. She took medication for allergies and migraines throughout her school years and earlier in her career when she held a university-based research position.

Her health stayed about the same until eight years ago, when she accepted a job that involved more teaching. At first, she found she was exhausted a lot of the time, and she attributed this to her early morning classes. But then she started to get headaches "that simply never went away." After a migraine that lasted for days, she went to her doctor at a health maintenance organization (HMO) and started what she refers to as the "great trek for a diagnosis." According to Gail, this was the time when she became "an active, continuous TMJ patient."

When talking from the perspective of the present, Gail attributes the dramatic increase in the severity of her headaches to the physical stress on her jaw caused by having to give classroom lectures. When she visited a physician, he linked the migraines to the stressful changes that had been going on in her life. He prescribed a commonly used medication as a prophylaxis for the migraines. At that time she accepted what the physician told her, thinking that it was just more of the same type of health problem she had had throughout her life, aggravated by the stress. She did not suspect that there could be something seriously wrong.

For approximately a year, Gail took the medications and consulted no other practitioners. In an attempt to cope with her headaches and manage stress, Gail started to meditate regularly.

> When I finally made my first breakthrough and just got my mind quiet, because it's real hard to do that, your mind's just babbling. What I noticed was there was clicking in my ear. I had no idea what that meant. But the first thing I noticed when my mind silenced, was that my body was in trouble.

Notwithstanding this incipient awareness of the body as the source of her problems, other experiences related to meditation aroused concerns that she might be headed toward serious psychological problems. She experienced what she refers to as "moments of intense inspiration" and "inspirational episodes":

> I didn't know what was happening. I would have these little episodes, not just of the pain, but . . . like a meditative state, like the state I would be in when I wanted to do a painting. But it would just suddenly come on me. Usually you've got to struggle, you've got to sit there to work at it, and it would just come.

She now explains these as "alpha waves all over my brain" which occurred because "I was so exhausted and my guard was down." At the time they started, however, she was not sure how to interpret them. On one hand, she thought of them as a source of religious and artistic inspiration through which she escaped her pain: "They were so sweet and so potent and so unexpected in the midst of all this misery that I wanted more of them. I wanted them all the time. And I wanted to learn what I needed to get them." On the other hand, they appeared to portend possible "psychotic episodes," "personality disintegration," or at the very least, "standard burnout and disillusionment": "I thought I was going nuts. And I thought I was having whopper migraines. I thought I was psychotic with continuous migraines."

The Search for Diagnosis

As a result of continued complaints about her migraines, her physician referred her to an allergist. She visited the allergist, who prescribed a weekly allergy shot and also found that Gail had a bad sinus infection and a maxillary polyp. After the infection was cleared up, she felt somewhat better, but the headaches continued. Referred to an ear, nose, and throat (ENT) specialist for a further examination of the polyp, which was found to be benign, Gail mentioned her migraines. The ENT specialist suggested her problems might be caused by TMJ. He gave her a cortisone shot and referred her to an oral surgeon. She felt the injection caused her jaw to move out of position: "My jaw started sort of flopping. You know, it didn't know where to go anymore. The place it had been stuck in, it had been moved out of, so now there was no new place to go." Asked about her initial reaction to TMJ, she replied:

> And I guess I figured it [TMJ] was like, you know, gum disease or something. I mean they would take care of it. I had no idea it was as complex, as difficult to understand, and as intractable to treat. I thought it was like the sinus infection. They give you some antibiotics. It goes away. I still believed that treatment worked.

During the six weeks between seeing the ENT physician and her appointment with the oral surgeon, Gail was in constant pain because of the dislocation of her jaw. Eating, lecturing, and even talking were extremely difficult. She lost weight. Although she continued to teach, she was unable to meet a deadline on a project for which she was hired as a consultant. At this point, she remembers beginning to feel anger against the HMO in particular and the medical profession in general because of the long lag between consultations. To Gail it seemed as if "they were just willing to let me sit there being in misery."

She finally met with the oral surgeon, only to endure a painful examination after which she left the office in more pain than when she arrived. The oral surgeon concluded that she did have TMJ but that it was only a muscular problem and there was therefore no reason to operate. Gail was informed that TMJ was a dental, not a medical, problem and told: "Sorry, we don't cover it, we don't pay for it, we don't treat it." A dentist was recommended.

Gail made two visits to this dentist, whom she describes as a "butcher."

On the second visit, he put in her first mouth appliance. The purpose of the appliance was to move the jaw back into its proper position, thereby reducing the stress on the muscles and eliminating the physiological basis for her pain. Wearing the appliance led to open sores and ultimately to a systemic infection. She called the dentist but was told that it would take time for her to get used to wearing the appliance and scheduled her for an appointment two weeks later. A week later, in great pain, she called again. After seeing her, the dentist called Gail's husband at his office to cancel her third appointment, saying she was no longer wanted as a patient as she was too demanding, and to request payment for the outstanding treatment charges.

In desperation, Gail and her husband picked another dentist through the telephone directory. He sent her to the HMO to get the systemic infection treated. Stating that the first appliance was all wrong, he constructed another one. He explained that there was a problem with her bite and her teeth weren't hitting right. This incorrect bite affected her joint, which in turn affected her muscles and led to her headaches. Gail feels that "of all the people I had talked to, he had the most compelling big picture." Yet at the same time, Gail recalls that "my husband is beginning to say, why should this guy's mouth appliance be any better than that guy's mouth appliance. You know, we're now moving into the realm where we don't really know how to evaluate."

Gail saw this dentist weekly for about two years. In addition to making three mouth appliances for her, the dentist also ground her teeth in an attempt to correct her bite. Although she initially felt positive about the treatment as it pulled her out of the "down cycle" she had been in previously, her health did not improve in the way she had hoped. As treatment continued and Gail did not get well, she started to ask questions about prognosis. The dentist suggested she return to the HMO to check if there was any arthritis in the jaw or any complicating neurological problems that could be impeding her progress. At this time, she says:

> I began to feel as though he didn't really have any answers in my specific case. That I was being viewed as a pest, because I would continue to inquire why the treatment was not just rolling right along like it was supposed to. . . . So, I began to lose a great deal of confidence.

Approximately eight months after her first visit to this dentist, Gail returned to the HMO requesting a referral to a neurologist. The neurologist diagnosed her problem as temporal lobe epilepsy and said that she had "small lesions" in her brain that were causing the "mildest form of epileptic attacks," which she interpreted as headaches. X rays were taken of her jaw, but no arthritic deterioration was found. She relates: "The neurologist was at this time not buying TMJ, he had his interest in epilepsy. So he was trying to prove that I didn't have TMJ." Gail now feels the diagnosis of epilepsy was made because she "fit the profile for women who are religious, who are artists, who like poetry, who have headaches, and I had had a trauma to the head." Yet, at the time of the diagnosis, when Gail was told her "inspirational episodes" were really epileptic seizures, she was "aghast to think that I had been misinterpreting physiological signals as something religious or in the realm of meditation." No CT scan was given at this time, and sleep-deprived electroencephalograms (EEGs)

> did not show anything that looked like epilepsy but did show a fairly sophisticated meditator. That is, I can make alpha waves at will. I can also make theta waves which are the very deepest, relaxing kinds of waves, so they found that. So then his theory was that I still really did have epilepsy and I was using my meditation as my own kind of drug.

Although Gail says she was not completely convinced that a diagnosis of epilepsy was warranted, she was willing to accept treatment in the hope that it would control the pain. Gail was prescribed six different medications to take daily. Shortly after starting this drug regimen,

> I had what we interpret as a seizure. I was sitting and writing something and I just sort of wasn't there for a while and when I came back my hand was sort of going back and forth so it looked like an EEG on paper where I had been writing, and just sort of trailed off. So I called and described that and he took it as an automatic confirmation of his diagnosis.

Although Gail had been told she would no longer experience the "inspirational episodes," she was unprepared for the side effects associated with the drugs. Of this period she states:

> I knew the pain was still there, but I was in such a fog that I wasn't complaining about it to the same degree. I think what people would tell you about that period is that what I was complaining about was that I wasn't myself anymore. I wasn't out of pain. I just didn't care anymore because I wasn't a human being. I was just a walking vegetable.

Her teaching and research suffered. She stopped accepting consulting jobs. She found herself unable to meditate. As a means of expression, Gail started to make drawings to represent her pain. She found this to be a much more powerful way of communicating the quality and intensity of pain than verbal expression. One drawing from this time is a self-portrait that Gail explained in the third person: "You can see she's got a chain around her jaw. She cannot see. She's so drugged, she's just looking out of this pain. And there's barbed wire running around her forehead as the bones, you know, implode."

After a year, Gail asked her primary-care physician to help her get off the epilepsy drugs because she was worse off than she was before treatment. The physician said that this was both inadvisable and dangerous. The physician referred Gail to a therapist trained in clinical psychology. Of this referral,

Gail said: "Now on the one hand I didn't like that because the point is that TMJ is not a psychological problem. But, given that my major complaint at the time was that I wasn't myself and I hated taking drugs, I think the therapist was a good idea."

Gail told the psychologist about the "eternal fog" that enveloped her throughout the day. Gail says: "She recognized that even though my sense of my pain was diminished, my sense of myself was also so diminished that it hadn't achieved anything." The psychologist said she had seen other women in a similar position, and it was her experience that temporal lobe epilepsy was a "garbage diagnosis" used when the patient was a woman and no other diagnosis seemed to fit. Against the advice of the physician, and without her guidance, the psychologist, over a period of seven months, helped Gail get off the drugs. Gail credits the psychologist with saving her life.

Around this time, one of Gail's friends married a neurologist. This neurologist cast further doubt on the epilepsy diagnosis. He felt that she had not been properly evaluated because her EEG was inconclusive and should have been followed up with a CT scan. He interpreted the "seizure" experienced while she was writing as a drug reaction caused by her attempts to lower her doses without supervision. He monitored Gail's progress as she came off the drugs and became more involved in what was happening. He later suggested a number of further diagnostic tests, which resulted in negative findings. She never had any seizure activity and states now that the epilepsy diagnosis "was another figment of their medical imagination." It was with this realization that she finally came to see TMJ as her central health problem.

The psychologist encouraged Gail to continue to deal with pain through meditation and art, suggesting that she try to make an image of the pain and figure out a way to release it. Gail described several of these images. One used the picture of herself with the chain around her jaw. She would imagine that someone with a wire cutter would cut the chain so that it would drop off and free her jaw. She displayed another drawing of a colorful bird whose talons are deeply embedded in a person's forehead, in the area where Gail feels the most pain. She would imagine the bird loosening its talons and flying away. In this way, her art became more than a way of expressing her pain: "It became a path that also actually blotted the pain out. It wasn't just a description of it. It was a way of getting rid of it." She developed other images that she used in meditation. A powerful image for her is to

imagine yourself as a tree, your feet digging down into the earth; roots come out from your toes. You feel the energy, the earth move up your body and when it gets to where it hurts, you imagine that you have leaves blossoming from you, and flowers. Each of those flowers is the pain, and I let the flowers drop off.

Throughout the time she was being treated for epilepsy, she continued to see the same dentist. His opinion was that epilepsy might be a complicating factor, but that she had real dental problems that couldn't be ignored. Explaining why she continued to receive treatment from him in spite of no improvement, she stated: "And remember I was pretty much a vegetable. I mean, I was on five different psychoactive drugs, so I was in no condition to make decisions about my own health care." Although she kept going to see him, she now says that although he diagnosed the problem correctly, his treatment was fundamentally incorrect:

> When that guy gave me the cortisone, I totally lost my bite. So I'm convinced that this dentist treated me when he really shouldn't have. That is, there should have been, maybe physical therapy, something to put me out of spasm before we rebuilt the bite based on an improper position that I was in from previous treatment. So that's why I think this treatment didn't work and was inappropriate, because it didn't take into account the violation. That he wasn't working with where I normally was. Of course I had no bite.

What finally led to discontinuing treatment with the dentist was an inability to continually pay for treatment. Since the initial consultation at the HMO three years earlier, Gail had incurred more than $15,000 in treatment costs.

The Search for Effective Treatment

For several months, Gail relied on art and meditation to control the pain, along with exercises she had been taught by the HMO's physical therapist. This therapist recommended Gail purchase a TENS (transcutaneous electrical stimulator) unit. Gail borrowed money to buy one. Gail also visited a local health spa regularly to soak her jaw in a whirlpool.

One day, while Gail was in the whirlpool, a woman came up to her and said she could tell Gail had TMJ, explaining she also used to visit the whirlpool to submerge her jaw. They exchanged stories, and the woman told Gail about the drawerful of mouth appliances she had at home, but also that she finally found relief with a dentist who specialized in building technologically sophisticated mouth appliances based on measurements of muscular activity.

Gail went to visit this new dentist, who requested an upfront payment of $1000 for construction of a new appliance. She again borrowed money. Although a bit skeptical, Gail signed a release form "saying I understood that I wasn't going to get well."

She saw this dentist twice a week for several months. The costs were high, although Gail reports a little improvement during this time. When the appliance broke and the dentist appeared unable to explain what was happening or to deal with the problem effectively, Gail decided to discontinue treatment.

Another treatment hiatus occurred, which was due to both lack of money and a continuing loss of confidence in the medical and dental professions' ability to treat TMJ. When money became available, her husband suggested she try a chiropractor, since physical therapy had previously provided some relief. She saw a chiropractor for six months, but without any real improvement in her condition. Looking back, Gail says:

> He said I definitely had it [TMJ], and that he had seen other TMJ patients. But then he also said to me, which I should have recognized as a sign—you know, you get to be a real sophisticated TMJ patient. By this time, I now know what all this stuff means. But he says, TMJ patients don't get well. They're not really my favorite patients because they don't get well, which I should have interpreted as, I do not know how to treat TMJ, I am a chiropractor. You got a bad back, I can help you.

Another six-month treatment hiatus followed. Gail felt her upper-body weakness and spasticity become noticeably worse. Her regular dentist, when she visited for a checkup, recommended a dentist associated with a TMJ specialty clinic. She made four visits to see him. On the fourth visit:

> At one point he adjusted the appliance. He put it in my mouth and when I stood up I heard a crack in my back and my limp became so exaggerated that it was like the opposite of Oral Roberts. You know, you go to Oral Roberts and you get healed. I went to this guy and came out limping, and I have been limping ever since.

When Gail complained that her back and pelvis had been affected by the appliance, the dentist replied there was no way these things could be related.

Gail returned to the HMO where sciatica was diagnosed and two weeks of bed rest was recommended. Completely disillusioned, Gail turned once more to the chiropractor in the hope that he would be able to help with the limp and back pain. The limp diminished over the five months of treatment, but for a year and a half Gail saw no one else for treatment.

Approximately a year before she was interviewed as part of this study, Gail joined the support group after reading a newspaper article. She joined out of "general desperation," hoping to learn about appropriate treatment through other people's experiences. Through the support group, she learned of a myotherapist who had taken up this profession because muscle therapy had successfully treated her own case of TMJ. For each visit, Gail received symptomatic relief that lasted several days. However, after seven visits the myotherapist suggested discontinuing treatment as she felt Gail's TMJ was not just a muscular problem, which myotherapy could treat, but that she had problems with her bite as well. She referred Gail to a TMJ dental specialist.

The initial examination by the TMJ specialist took two hours. His interest in Gail's past history with TMJ and the attention paid to the concerns she raised struck Gail as very humane. The TMJ specialist also told Gail that he was a TMJ sufferer who had trained in this specialty because of his own experiences. In many respects, his explanation of TMJ was consistent with what she had been told previously, but he also provided new insights:

> He did give me new information which I didn't know, which was that your cranial bones move. Before that everyone else I had always talked to assumed that it was just the mandible that is mobile in TMJ patients and the skull stays stable, and it's not that way at all. . . . He also said that the disease had progressed enough in my case that it wasn't just my head anymore, that was throwing everything off, but my pelvis had been shifting for so long ever since that other guy gave me the limp. My pelvis had been doing such a job of trying to compensate that it was now totally off too. So I was sort of broken at both ends. So that in my particular case we couldn't just treat it from the neck up, as though the rest of me hadn't been trying to compensate for it underneath the shifting cranium for seven years.

His explanation provided Gail with a model that integrated the different problems she had experienced over the years. It also provided a rationale for treatment. The TMJ specialist was able to arrange for most of his expenses to be covered by medical insurance. He also suggested TMJ chiropractic treatment to complement the mouth appliances that he would build.

Gail started to visit the chiropractor, who specializes in what he calls sacral-occipital therapy. He does adjustments to her cranium and mandible, both externally and from within her mouth, along with standard chiropractic care for the rest of her body.

Gail has seen both of these practitioners weekly for the past seven months. She sees a big difference between how she felt when starting treatment and how she feels at present:

> He [the chiropractor] does strength testing. On my intake interview I could press twenty-five pounds on my right hand and eight pounds on my left. I can now press forty pounds on my right hand and twenty pounds on my left. In terms of my pelvis, the limp is now almost entirely gone. I have more pain-free days. I sleep better. I have more residual strength and resistance. My artwork has drastically improved. I can show you when I started treatment and you can see it in my drawings. And my husband says it's not like living with the same person . . . this is much more like who I used to be than it is like who I was under all the drug therapy.

Gail describes herself as "forty percent improved." Also, whereas before she would often have pain episodes lasting five or six days, she is now usually able to terminate one by visiting the chiropractor. When she started treatment, the TMJ specialist said that in about two to three years she could have "a life again," although he also cautioned that she will always have to be careful not to overstress her jaw and its structural balance. She remains hopeful but unsure how much more they will be able to help her. This is, however, the first time she feels her problem is being directly addressed.

The Body in Pain

Initially, Gail saw her body as an object to be fixed through medical treatment: "I thought some man in a white coat was going to find an answer and make me better." Her narrative recounts instances to the contrary, when interactions with medical practitioners led to increased physical suffering. Of her current treatment, Gail says, "It is a new thing for me to actually have appropriate treatment, where when you leave you feel better." Gail feels that medical practitioners often fail to recognize that she and other patients are human beings who are suffering and in pain: "It's a terrible thing to fall into the hands of the whitecoats. It is. Because they treat you like a body that's all cut up into little pieces and they never look at you as a whole person."

Gail describes the present condition of her body as "broken," "vulnerable," and in need of "love and attention." Gail sees "illness as a way our bodies talk to us" and says it is important to "not cut off that language by dulling it with drugs." When taking the epilepsy drugs, Gail lost the ability to communicate with her body. Since coming off the drugs, pain has led Gail to an increased awareness of her embodied state:

> I think of pain as extended consciousness of your body. I think that most normal people . . . are not at all aware of their bodies. . . . So that in some ways, pain restores us to what every aborigine or tribal person in the ancient world used to have, which is a sense of their internal universe . . . they were much more in tune to where their body is in their environment. If pain is the only way that a modern person can be taught to re-experience their body, then I can see it has a sort of educational stage, but not necessarily a terminal end point to my life.

When asked what was her body trying to tell her, Gail replied:

> It was saying, we hurt, and you're not paying attention. You're trying to live this disembodied life of the mind and you haven't attended to yourself as a person. So it told me to stop acting like super scholar and start living as a human being and that was a good thing to hear. So I trust my body's wisdom.

Although Gail feels she is improving, she likens herself to a recovering alcoholic: "you're alcohol free, the problem's gone . . . but you have to live in balance if you want to keep it under control." An important part of this is maintaining an awareness of the limitations of her body and a self-conscious attitude about eating properly, getting enough rest, and avoiding things that may overstress her body physically.

Mind and Pain

Although TMJ has led to greater awareness of her body, development of her skills in meditation has taught her that the mind can exert a powerful influence on the perception of pain. This is not always easy: "What you are trying to do is totally blank your mind and totally forget about your

body. . . . But I'm in a body that won't be forgotten; it hurts too much."
Meditation and concentration on her art have become a means through
which Gail is able to escape her body and its pain:

> Art. . . I sometimes think that what I'm going for is disembodiment in the
> sense that a loss of. . . the consciousness of continuous pain. When I do my
> artwork or when I'm intensely focused in meditation or anything, I go out of
> myself. I'm not just bound by my body.

Meditation, however, has become more than a way to blot out pain; it has
become a way to heal the body. Gail sees the relationship between mind and
body as one in which the mind can promote physical well-being. She is currently experimenting, using visual images of her jaw moving into a correct
position. She thinks that

> the relationship between the mind and body is profound and powerful because
> I have such an effect on altering my own pain and my sensations of pain. I can't
> help but know that the mind is involved in this. During the time when I haven't
> had treatment I have tended to focus intensely on what I could do through
> meditation. And so ever since I've emerged from the drugs, I've been a very
> active partner in my own cure.

Part of the reason Gail is enthusiastic about the dentist and chiropractor
who are currently treating her is that, in marked contrast to the health-care
professionals she previously consulted, they respect her need to meditate and
what she feels she can achieve through it.

Gail views TMJ as essentially a physical problem: "Pain causes stress,
stress doesn't cause pain. . . . I'm not going to take the rap for having a lousy
personality when all I need is to have my cranium adjusted." Though Gail
acknowledges that psychosocial stress can exacerbate her physical problems,
she sees it as a contributing but not causative factor and is quick to point out
that physical or "biomechanical" stress is more likely to cause ill health. At
the same time, she recognizes the appeal of psychosocial explanations, for
both physician and patient, when no physical basis for illness can be found.

> The brain wants to make order out of what happens to us. It wants to have
> experience make sense. And we'll find a way to make it make sense, no matter
> what kind of mental gymnastics we have to go through. And see, that's why
> we're so susceptible to this psychological model of TMJ, because we're doing
> it ourselves.

Indeed, there are times in Gail's narrative when she actively considered or
accepted psychosocial explanations for her pain. The first was when she took
up her teaching position and her headaches worsened. Initially, she assumed
they were linked to the stress of starting this new job. When the HMO physician suggested the same thing, she had no problem accepting this explanation. As time went by without resolution of her problems, this explanation

became more elaborate. Gail felt that some of the other faculty members did not approve of some of the controversial topics, such as feminism and homosexual rights, she sometimes used in classroom discussions. Thus,

> when I got my first appliance, I thought this is what they want, I'm muzzled. . . . I felt that I had been wounded in the very part of me that was dangerous to the existing culture in which I work. And so, I found myself a symbolic illness to express what they were doing to me intellectually and my body found a way to work that out.

In addition, the "inspirational episodes" seemed to presage a mental breakdown.

As time went on and Gail's problems worsened, however, the psychological approach no longer seemed appropriate. Gail's life up to the start of her illness had included other troublesome experiences, which led her to conclude that it did not make sense "for somebody as strong as me to crumble just because I was in a new setting. That's not at all what we would have predicted based on any of my past life experiences." Thus, although a psychologically based explanation seemed plausible initially, as the illness continued, Gail grew to distrust "cute psychological explanations" and became suspicious of "people who give psychological reasons for physical problems."

Gail also believes that the attribution of a psychological cause for TMJ commonly occurs.

> Some people still think of TMJ as so much a psychological complex of problems that maybe they [the insurance company] will cover it and maybe they won't. . . . And it was, it was so frustrating. It's so frustrating to be legitimately ill and have people treating you as though you're faking it, or you're just another crazy female. Or, you could be well if you wanted to, you just need to be more positive about things.

Citing statistics that demonstrate that more women than men seek medical care for symptoms of TMJ, Gail suggests that this brings out a bias in the medical profession "to assume that a woman is more open to psychological problems, that she is not reporting something that is physically real, but she is hypochondriacal."

Growing through Pain

Although embittered about her interactions with medical professionals, the lived experience of illness and pain has had profound implications on how Gail sees her life plan. In spite of the misery she has endured, she says:

> If somebody came to me and said, would you take the last seven years, given where your head is now, or would you rather not have had those seven years and not know what you know now, and not have trained yourself in them, I would

still choose what has happened to me. That is how extraordinary my experiences have been and how re-creational they've been in the sense that I have a freedom to be a whole person now that I never did before I meditated.

Pain and TMJ has changed the way she sees her life and the world:

My experience of being in constant pain affects everything. How I think about my past. How I think about my future. The joy that I have when I'm drawing, sculpting. It's in the face of the pain, you know. It's like a shadow that throws the other parts of my life into brighter contrast. You see my brights are brighter, cause I have this darkness hovering all around the edges . . . the world has become a more precious and beautiful place—because I really see it.

Before TMJ, Gail describes her life as firmly based in the academic world. In school, both she and her advisors saw her as a potential leader in her field who was "expected to go out and set the world on fire." Through pain she has come to realize that there are "bigger things than deadlines in this world and bigger things than status."

Gail's life now "revolves around meditation and art." Through her art, Gail hopes to help people who are not in pain understand what it is like to be in pain:

I want my art to help people know that there is a way through their pain. In other words, my art explicates where I've been in pain. I call it the land of shadow. I say there's some of us who walk in shadow and we learn that. And everybody's going to encounter it sometime. Somebody you love is going to die or you're going to get sick. So I feel as though those of us who walk in shadow every day, and find a path through it and try to live normally with some integrity and some hope, that we have something very special to say to normals, which is what I call people who don't have pain, and to the whitecoats, which is what I call the medical establishment.

For Gail, suffering from chronic pain is like "having a sword hanging over you." She is unable to predict how she will feel the next day or even the next hour. This has led to a greater appreciation of time, especially of times when her pain is less. She says she has become a more flexible person and more understanding of what she used to think of as "failings" in others. By teaching people through her art what it means to have pain, Gail hopes people will also realize what is truly important in life:

And all these people in pain . . . all these people with aches and all these people suffering. We walk in different dimensions. We have access to different experiences, different knowledge. And there are so many of us, too. What would happen if we all knew what it really meant and we all lived as if it really mattered, which it does. We could help the normals and the whitecoats both. We could help them see that they're wasting the precious moments of their lives, if they would look at us who don't have it. I'm convinced only sick people know what health is. And they know it by its very loss. I see people all the time who walk across the street, or pick up a bag of groceries and never give it a second thought. I pick up a bag of groceries and don't feel too bad when I do it, I rejoice. It's a whole different aspect. . . . When I see my students worrying about trivial matters, I just laugh. C'mon folks, the real thing here is to live the days you have and live them well. Furiously. It's the only revenge you've got.

Consistent with the changes in her life plan, the goals Gail has set for herself have also been reevaluated: "My major goal is not that I write books and everyone says 'Hurray, isn't she smart, isn't she brilliant' but that people look at my painting and say 'God, what suffering, but what hope.'"

Gail has been able to transform her pain from seemingly meaningless suffering that isolated her from others to something that gives meaning to her life: "I can't help but feel like. . . not that there's a purpose to my pain, but that I haven't let it triumph. I've made it into something else. I've made it into a way to make connections to people."

COMPARING THE NARRATIVES

As examples of narrative construction, the two stories reported here are unique. Yet they share similarities in structure and content, reflecting the challenges posed by the "ontological assault" of chronic pain and shared experiences with the health-care system in a North American cultural setting.

At the level of structure, both narratives follow the outline proposed earlier: from genesis, to major disruption, to the search for a diagnosis, to search for appropriate treatment. This prototypical narrative structure, with its focus on treatment, reflects salient features of the health-seeking process in North American society (Chrisman 1977) for conditions, such as TMJ, which are difficult both to diagnose and to treat.

All the individuals interviewed had received and almost all had accepted, at least for the time being, a diagnosis of TMJ as an explanation for at least some of their difficulties. As the narratives are stories in progress, there is no common resolution for the final stage. Nevertheless, there appear to be three general patterns. Some individuals were still searching for effective treatment. For others, even though they are still suffering, the search had, for the moment at least, stopped for reasons ranging from financial constraints to despair at ever finding help. The third pattern, exemplified by the two narratives presented here, occurs when individuals report a lessening of their physical problems because of the care they currently receive and thus no longer actively search for alternative help.

Individuals represented by the third pattern reported receiving treatment that was sensitive to their experiences and congruent with their explanatory model of TMJ. A sense of control over TMJ is also present in these narratives (see Brody 1980; Cassel 1982:641; Eisenberg 1981:245). Often, a current practitioner is seen to provide a key element of the explanatory model, which is then used to reconstruct past experiences and provide a basis for future treatment actions. Molly's explanatory model was not complete until the homeopathic physician helped her to interpret the initially frightening reversal of symptoms. For Gail, it was her current dentist who explained how a problem primarily localized in her jaw could lead to symptoms throughout her body. Both Molly and Gail feel that their current practitioners are responsive to their needs, and both portray them as more humane than other practitioners consulted earlier in their treatment history. Unlike others consulted, these practitioners provide external validation for their pain and dysfunction and the wide range of symptoms they experience. Both Molly and Gail feel they have achieved some control over their illness: Molly through repeated visits for treatment; Gail through treatment and her own personal methods of art and meditation.

Yet it must be stressed that for chronic pain.sufferers what constitutes an acceptable explanation and treatment is subject to revision. Whether Gail and Molly would make similar statements about their explanatory models, their practitioners, and the degree of control achieved over the illness, in the context of a repeat interview at a later time, remains an open question. As the view of the past is shaped by the present, the view of the present from the perspective of the future will be shaped by that future.

At the level of content, the narratives also address similar issues. The challenges of chronic pain are the same for both, although the responses differ. These challenges include questions raised about the authenticity of the pain experience, changes in the relationship between self and body as a result of illness, and revising the life plan in light of the disruptive effects of TMJ.

All individuals interviewed mentioned being confronted with the view that their pain was caused by stress in their lives. In the narratives, two models of the stress process were discussed, though certainly not all individuals adopted a social stress explanation. In the first, a person under stress has a physical response, such as grinding the teeth or clenching the jaw, which eventually leads to TMJ through continual muscle spasms or changes in jaw position. This model of stress formed part of a number of narratives and was not seen as challenging the reality of pain. Here, stress contributes to abnormalities in the temporomandibular joint, and it is these abnormalities that are the actual cause of the pain and dysfunction.

The contrasting view of stress excludes the possibility of an organic basis for pain. Both the cause of pain and the potential for the control of pain are based in the psychological response of the individual to stressful experiences. The failure of an individual to improve in spite of treatment is attributable to inadequacies of the individual and not to inadequacies in treatment (see Marbach and Lipton 1987; Kotarba 1983; Kotarba and Seidel 1984; Lennon et al. 1989). This second model of stress challenges the integrity of the self

(Eisenberg 1981:245), and the common reaction in the narratives was a rejection of this model, at least as the primary cause of TMJ, followed by a continued search for validation from other health-care providers. Molly's story is an example: she repudiates all suggestions that the stress in her life is causing her physical problems and continues to visit a variety of practitioners until her illness is identified as TMJ. In order to keep practitioners from labeling her problem as psychogenic, she develops a strategy based on the selective telling of symptoms and treatment history when first consulting a potential healer.

Nevertheless, many individuals interviewed said at some point they considered mental stress as a possible cause of their problems. This reflects the popularity of the stress concept as an explanation for illness in North American culture. However, this tended to happen early, before TMJ was a serious disruption in their lives and before many practitioners were consulted. This can be seen in Gail's story: she initially accepts an interpretation of her headaches as caused by the stress of taking up a demanding new job. However, as the pain worsens in spite of her efforts to meditate to counter the effects of stress, the stress hypothesis becomes untenable. Further suggestions that her problems are caused by stress lead to dissatisfaction, disillusionment, and anger directed toward health-care providers. Those telling other narratives would often accept the idea that stress could amplify their physical symptoms, but insisted there was a physical problem that was primary. When faced with a stress interpretation without an organic basis, individuals usually continued to seek out additional practitioners until a diagnosis of TMJ was made. It is somewhat ironic that as people become less receptive to purely psychological interpretations of their pain, health-care providers become more likely to apply psychogenic interpretations and to view their clients as "problem" patients.

The second challenge is that of adjusting to limitations of the body that develop as a consequence of TMJ. Illness forces an awareness of the body as separate from self. Perhaps the most common response to the body in illness, exemplified to an extreme by Molly's narrative, is to see the body both as an object in need of being fixed and as an obstacle that constrains and opposes self (Gadow 1980). In this view, illness has the "character of insurgence: the body rebels, the self is thwarted" (Gadow 1980:180). For Molly, the rebellious body comes to be controlled through treatment. In Gail's narrative, this view of the body as object is also present. It predominates during the early period of her illness when she hopes someone in a white coat will fix her jaw, but it never entirely goes away. Over time, the dominant response to her body changes so that she comes to see it as a "being in its own right" (Gadow 1980:180) and a source of values and knowledge for how to live her life. For Gail, it is her body and her experience with pain that lead to the reevaluation of her life-style and her life goals.

Both Molly and Gail's responses to their bodies are the catalysts for changes in the life plan. As their responses to their bodies are quite different, so are their revised life plans. Molly essentially comes to adopt her sickness as a career in an attempt to fix and exert control over her body. Two components are essential to the development of this revised life plan: the external validation of a structural imbalance by health-care providers as well as procedures for correcting this imbalance. Molly's response to illness before these two components are in place is simply to adjust her level of functioning to reflect physical constraints. The development of the revised life plan provides a sense of meaning and control that was missing in earlier stages of her illness. For Gail, the revised life does not depend on the validation of the illness by others. Indeed, her life plan had changed before discovering her current practitioners. Rather, the revision to Gail's life plan is the outcome of a process of exploration centering on meditation and art. It is through meditation and art that Gail comes to understand her body and achieve control over her illness.

For both Molly and Gail, the revised life plans do not completely supplant pre-illness life plans; they assert both the continuity of self and the changes in self through illness. Although Molly stops working, she still receives income in the form of disability payments. Her central identity as wife and mother is enhanced rather than diminished through the revision, as she now has more time and renewed energy to spend with her family. Gail, although firmly committed to developing her art, continues to teach and does not intend to give up her academic career. She has, however, given up external consulting activities even though these projects provided additional sources of income. The revised life plan allows her to direct much of her limited energy to those activities she now finds meaningful while providing a justification for not working incessantly to increase her number of publications and status in her field.

What comes across very strongly in these narratives is that Molly and Gail maintain their sense of identity in spite of their suffering and the repeated questioning of the authenticity of their pain. For Gail, getting off the epilepsy drugs was a means of self-preservation in the most basic sense. It is against those practitioners whose statements and other actions were perceived as a threat to self that Gail and Molly direct the bulk of their anger.

Drawing on the particular experiences of two individuals, this chapter has attempted to identify similarities in structure and content that characterize the illness narratives of the participants in this study. To understand the impact of illness and treatment on a person's life, it is necessary to develop an understanding of the narrative context. Although it is impossible to anticipate a particular narrative, it is possible to anticipate some of the concerns they will address (Brody 1987:192). By identifying similarities in structure and themes while representing diversity in individual response to TMJ, the approach described here takes a middle ground, somewhere between the elaboration of case studies as singular examples in their own right and the reductionism of quality of life and pain questionnaires.

ACKNOWLEDGMENTS

I would like to acknowledge the involvement of Byron Good and Karen Stephenson as co-investigators. We thank the individuals who graciously agreed to be interviewed. I would also like to thank Leon Eisenberg for his help in getting this project underway. Mary-Jo DelVecchio Good, Byron Good, Arthur Kleinman, James Lipton, Karen Stephenson, Linda Hunt, Robert Whitmore, and participants in the weekly medical anthropology seminar at Harvard University made helpful suggestions on earlier versions of this paper. This project was supported by internal funds from the Department of Social Medicine and Health Policy, Harvard Medical School, and by a University of Manitoba Research Grant. The data were collected while the author was a research fellow in the Clinically Relevant Medical Anthropology Training Program in the Department of Social Medicine, Harvard Medical School, codirected by Dr. A. Kleinman and Dr. B. Good (NIMH Grant No. 5-T32-MH18006). During the analysis and write-up phase, the author received support from the National Health Research Development Program of Canada through a Scholar Award.

NOTE

1. Of course, illness occurs within a social setting, and another area of shared content is how relationships with others, such as family, co-workers, and friends are seen as affected by the narrator's experience with chronic illness. There is, however, little mention of this topic in this chapter, although such information was variably discussed in the interviews. In part the decision to omit this topic is due to space constraints, but it also reflects a concern with maintaining confidentiality. I felt the narrative construction approach was not an appropriate vehicle for exploring these issues.

REFERENCES CITED

Berger, J., and J. Mohr
   1967   *A fortunate man: The story of a country doctor.* London: Allen Lane, Penguin Press.
Berger, P., and T. Luckman
   1966   *The social construction of reality.* Garden City, N.Y.: Doubleday.
Brody, H.
   1980   *Placebos and the philosophy of medicine.* Chicago: University of Chicago Press.

1987   *Stories of sickness.* New Haven, Conn., and London: Yale University Press.

Bury, M.
1982   Chronic illness as biographical disruption. *Sociology of Health and Illness* 4:167–182.

Cassel, E. J.
1982   The nature of suffering and the goals of medicine. *New England Journal of Medicine* 306:639–645.

Chrisman, N.
1977   The health seeking process: An approach to the natural history of an illness. *Culture, Medicine and Psychiatry* 1:351–377.

De Boever, J. A.
1979   Functional disturbances of the temporomandibular joint. In *Temporomandibular joint function and dysfunction*, G. A. Zarb and G. E. Carlsson, eds., 193–214. Copenhagen: Munksgaard.

Eisenberg, L.
1981   The physician as interpreter: Ascribing meaning to the illness experience. *Comprehensive Psychiatry* 22:239–248.

Fabrega, H., and P. Manning
1972   Disease, illness and deviant careers. In *Theoretical perspectives on deviance*, R. A. Scott and J. D. Douglas, eds. New York: Basic Books.

Franks, A. S. T.
1964   The social character of temporomandibular joint dysfunction. *The Dental Practitioner* 15:94–100.

Fricton, J. R., R. Kroening, D. Haley, and R. Siegert
1985   Myofascial pain syndrome of the head and neck: A review of clinical characteristics of 164 patients. *Oral Surgery* 60:615–623.

Gadow, S.
1980   Body and self: A dialectic. *Journal of Medicine and Philosophy* 5:172–185.

Griffiths, R. H.
1983   Report of the president's conference on the examination, diagnosis and management of temporomandibular disorders. *Journal of the American Dental Association* 106:75–77.

Kelley, M. P.
1986   The subjective experience of chronic disease: Some implications for the management of ulcerative colitis. *Journal of Chronic Diseases* 39:653–666.

Kleinman, A.
1980   *Patients and healers in the context of culture.* Berkeley, Los Angeles, London: University of California Press.
1986   Illness meanings and illness behavior. In *Illness behavior: A multidisciplinary model*, S. McHugh and M. Vallis, eds., 149–160. New York: Plenum Press.
1988   *The illness narratives: Suffering, healing and the human condition.* New York: Basic Books.

Kotarba, J. A.
1983   *Chronic pain: Its social dimensions.* Beverly Hills, Calif.: Sage Publications.

Kotarba, J. A., and J. V. Seidel
1984   Managing the problem pain patient: Compliance or social control. *Social*

Science and Medicine 19:1393–1400.

Lennon, M. C., B. G. Link, J. J. Marbach, and B. P. Dohrenwend
  1989   The stigma of chronic facial pain and its impact on social relationships. *Social Problems* 36:117–134.

Marbach, J. J., and J. A. Lipton
  1978   Aspects of illness behavior in patients with facial pain. *Journal of the American Dental Association* 96:630–638.
  1987   Biopsychosocial factors of the temporomandibular pain dysfunction syndrome: Relevance to restorative dentistry. *Dental Clinics of America* 31:473–486.

Moss, R. A., J. Garrett, and J. F. Chiodo
  1982   Temporomandibular joint dysfunction and myofascial pain dysfunction syndromes: Parameters, etiology, and treatment. *Psychological Bulletin* 92:331–346.

Murphy, R. F.
  1987   *The body silent.* New York: Henry Holt.

Nardi, B.
  1983   Goals in reproductive decision making. *American Ethnologist* 10:697–715.

National Institute for Dental Research
  1990   Broadening the scope: Long-range research plan for the nineties. Bethesda, Md.: National Institute of Health.

Parsons, T.
  1951   *The social system.* New York: Free Press.

Pellegrino, E. D.
  1979   Toward a reconstruction of medical morality: The primacy of the act of profession and the fact of illness. *Journal of Medicine and Philosophy* 4:32–56.

Quinn, N., and D. Holland
  1987   Culture and cognition. In *Cultural models in language and thought*, D. Holland and N. Quinn, eds., 3–40. Cambridge: Cambridge University Press.

Reif, L.
  1973   Managing a life with chronic disease. *American Journal of Nursing* 73:261–264.

Sacks, O.
  1985   *The man who mistook his wife for a hat.* New York: Summit Books.

Strauss, A. L., and B. G. Glaser
  1975   *Chronic illness and the quality of life.* St. Louis: Mosby.

Turner, B. S.
  1984   *The body and society: Explorations in social theory.* Oxford: Basil Blackwell.

Von Korff, Michael, et al.
  1988a   Temporomandibular disorders: Variation in clincial practice. *Medical Care* 26:307–314.

Von Korff, Michael, et al.
  1988b   An epidemiological comparison of pain complaints. *Pain* 32:173–183.

Wiener, C.
  1975   The burden of rheumatoid arthritis: Tolerating the uncertainty. *Social Science and Medicine* 9:97–104.

Williams, G.
   1984   The genesis of chronic illness: Narrative reconstruction. *Sociology of
           Health and Illness* 6:175–200.
   1987   Disablement and the social context of daily activity. *International Disabil-
           ity Studies* 9:97–102.
Williams, G., and P. H. N. Wood
   1986   Common-sense beliefs about illness: A mediating role for the doctor. *The
           Lancet* 27:1435–1437.

CHAPTER SIX

"After a While No One Believes You": Real and Unreal Pain

Jean E. Jackson

I disagreed with their big philosophies . . . Dr. V said pain isn't physical—you can't set pain down, look at it. But I said, "Well, I see pain as part of the workings of the body, like electricity. You can't see electricity, but you grab the end of a wire in a machine, and it'll hurt you."

Comments such as this from patients at a chronic pain treatment center in New England (here referred to as the Commonwealth Pain Center, or CPC[1]) reveal a concern with how "real" or "unreal" their pain is seen to be. One might initially think that the contrast between "real" and "unreal" is simple: real is organic, physical pain, whereas unreal is "all in your head" pain—imaginary, mental, emotional, psychosomatic. My research revealed that this contrast, while very significant in itself, also contains a more elaborate classification system, for "unreal" is actually a cover term for a set of rather fuzzy and complicated notions. Although some of the confusion patients report about their pain problem arises from a simple misapprehension of medical terminology (e.g., *malingering*, *psychosomatic*), most ambiguity is due to: (1) the nature of pain itself (its invisibility, its subjectivity, its challenge to Western mind/body dualism), (2) contradictory ideas about responsibility for one's condition, (3) stigma and demoralization, and (4) the CPC's unusual treatment program.

The social context of treatment at the CPC, involving intensive interaction, results in patients creating new intersubjective meanings of pain during their month or more of participation in the unit's therapeutic community. Note that while the expression "real pain" is heard a great deal at the CPC, no patient or staff member uses the phrase "unreal pain" with any frequency. Although CPC patients see their problem in terms of "real" pain due to "real" causes,[2] the unspoken presence of "unreal pain" in many interactions there requires that we understand what it means if we want to fathom pain sufferers' talk about pain and the challenges to this "pain talk" mounted by fellow patients and CPC staff.

This chapter is not an analysis of patients' narratives about pain, nor does it examine talk per se. Since I found that patients report confusion, or at best a partial understanding of their own and others' pain problems, I draw on "bits of talk" from many patients to illustrate how this talk feeds into the overall discourse about pain at the CPC. Bits of talk are presented in mosaic, rather than linear, fashion to convey the flavor of the often quite inchoate discourse taking place, illustrating the chapter's main point: that confusion, some of it the product of a process of mystification of pain by CPC staff, plays a major role in constituting the discourse about pain in settings like the CPC.

This chapter also takes a *patient-focused, experiential* approach. I eschew clinical language where possible because language used by patients themselves, arising out of their own comprehensions and perceptions, is a superior guide for understanding their experience.

From a phenomenological perspective, the distinction between pain behavior, the experience of pain, and the emotional states accompanying pain, such as suffering or demoralization, is highly ambiguous (see Jackson, n.d.2). Furthermore, definitions of chronic pain provided in the clinical literature seldom establish clarity and agreement: although one author's typology according to symptoms or cause may appear tidy, taken as a whole, the literature on chronic pain is confused. In the conclusions to this paper, I suggest that the ambiguity of the "reality" of pain not only reflects the nature of the pain experience and its obdurate resistance to objectification and treatment, but that this ambiguity is systematically heightened as a modality of treatment at the CPC in which pain is mystified as a means to breaking down the mental constructs patients have about pain which resist change.

Research was carried out at the CPC from February 1986 to February 1987. In eight months of participant observation there, I observed 173 resident patients. I also conducted 196 interviews with 136 patients (60 of whom were interviewed twice) and interviewed 20 staff members as well. The main focus of the research was an investigation of "cognitive restructuring" in patients—to see how changes in thinking about pain were correlated with self-reports about improvement.

Sources of Confusion about "Real" Pain

Sources that create ambiguity in and confound the meaning of "real" pain are found in everyday common-sense encounters with pain, in medical and clinical experiences in the treatment of pain, and in the varieties of authoritative themes generated by pain researchers. Pain is invisible. We infer the presence of pain in someone else indirectly, from observation (e.g., a broken leg) or through communication from the sufferer—pain behavior. Pain behavior can be an attempt to communicate the experience of pain or the expression of affects—of suffering, of demoralization, of other feelings and ideas associated with the pain experience. Indeed, separating "the pain experience" from other experiences accompanying pain, but somehow viewed apart from "real" pain itself, is a demanding, perhaps impossible, task.

Most authorities on pain define pain as a subjective experience, a feeling we cannot observe or measure directly.[3] This means that one must be conscious to have pain: during an operation the anesthesia, if properly administered, eliminates pain by making the patient unconscious. When asked what pain is, staff members at the CPC sometimes reply that "pain is what the patient says it is."[4] This highlights pain's subjectivity, although such a phenomenologically based definition is virtually useless for most experimental or medical purposes. Hilbert (1984) maintains that grasping the notion of chronic pain—unending pain—is impossible because a key semantic feature of "pain" is the notion of temporality.[5] Indeed, a parsimonious, albeit understated, definition of hell is severe chronic pain.[6]

While pain in general is seen as a biologically useful process, chronic pain is defined as any continuing pain that has lost its biological function (Bonica 1976:11; Black 1979:34). When a pain appears, it usually indicates nociception (the onset of a provoking or harmful condition)—a symptom rather than a disease, a "normal" indication of something abnormal. Any chronic pain whose underlying pathology is unclear (which is the case for many patients at the CPC) thus confounds our common-sense notions of disease and health. Pain centers such as the CPC advocate conceiving chronic pain as the problem rather than an indication of a problem, but this is a novel idea. These new pain centers, and the language, philosophy, international organizations, journals, and meetings that are associated with them, can be seen as an instance of the cultural construction of a disease. While CPC staff and other pain specialists would agree that pain always "serves a function," in many cases this function is not considered useful or authentic. Hence, the discourse on chronic pain frequently becomes a moral discourse, evident not only at the CPC and at similar pain centers, but also in the medical literature. In a very important sense, the primary meaning connoted by "real" pain is one of legitimacy—pain one is entitled to because one has in no way brought it upon oneself. Insofar as chronic pain serves an illegitimate function, it is itself illegitimate.

Clinicians' understandings of pain are complex and varied, depending in part on their medical specialty and on the specifics of a given case. Definition would seem to be crucial. Yet, while there is agreement regarding the differences between acute and chronic pain (Pinsky 1975:383; Bokan, Ries, and Katon 1981:331), the literature reveals significant disagreement about chronic pain and chronic pain syndrome.[7] In general, the clinicians' debate focuses on the extent to which chronic pain is due to psychogenic, rather than physical, causes, and the consequent implications for treatment.

One might expect the research literature on pain to provide enlighten-ment. Unfortunately, the abundance of definitions, classifications, and dis-agreements contained in the writings of pain experts enlightens us best on just how difficult defining and understanding chronic pain is. For example, *benign* chronic pain is distinguished from *malign* chronic pain (i.e., caused by a malignancy), signaling that the source of the pain probably will not kill the person.[8] But from the point of view of the sufferer of intractable pain, *benign* is hardly a satisfactory descriptor, and for this reason other experts disagree with this usage (Bonica 1985:xxxiii). Another descriptor is *intractable*.[9] However, Cademenos (1981:77) maintains that *intractable* is something of a medical excuse, since it simply refers to forms of pain which cannot be oper-ationally defined or verified. Authors also disagree about classifications of psychogenic pain. For example, Pilowski (1978:212) shows why the dif-ferentiation between conversion and hypochondriacal reactions is unsatisfac-tory and also maintains that the distinction between "genuine" and "false" pain is spurious (1978:206). Fordyce criticizes "physiological" versus "psychological" and "organic" versus "functional" divisions because they "connote a Cartesian dualism and should have been discarded long ago" (1978:52; see also Menges 1981:89). Black classifies "chronic pain" as psychogenic and uses the phrase "recurrent acute pain" (in fact, also a form of chronic pain) for organic pain (1979:34; also see Agnew, Crue, Pinsky 1979). And while it would seem that a behaviorally focused program would automatically imply an assumption of psychogenic pain, Bonica and Fordyce (1974:311) say that to argue that all patients in a behavioral program had psychogenic pain would beg the question, since each patient had at some time been diagnosed as having some medically based pain.

A majority of pain centers assume a somewhat psychologically minded stance toward chronic pain and reject basing decisions about treatment sole-ly on conventional biomedical findings from X rays and CT scans. Words such as "habit" and "motivation" frequently appear in the literature report-ing on research carried out in such centers, as do acknowledgments of the impact on the patient of psychosocial factors such as family support. But pain centers appear to differ a great deal in the degree of psychological em-phasis and type of psychological intervention; for example, some stress depth psychology, while others favor behavioral approaches.

Some pain-center programs focus on pain *behavior* so exclusively that they seem unconcerned with pain itself: if there were no pain behavior, they say, there would be no pain problem, and thus their goal is to eliminate the pain behavior (see Fordyce 1978:54). While many clinicians take exception to this notion, it *is* clear that many greatly admire those patients who "suffer with dignity"—that is, quietly, with a minimum of pain behavior. Marcus states that improved function is what matters, not whether the pain is the same or less (in Schaeffer 1983:25). Other pain specialists stress the need to reduce the pain experience itself. Some link the two goals, commenting that an acceptance of psychological causes can lead to feeling better: "often the apparent acceptance of the diagnosis at 5, 6, or 7 weeks post-admission coincided with a dramatic reduction in pain" (Sarno 1976:149).

Black notes that when physicians repeat failed diagnostic procedures, which seek organic causes, rather than ones trying to assess the patient as a totality with social and economic factors taken into consideration, eventually the patient will feel there is no objective basis and will be "forced to conclude he has some sort of mental problem" (1979:40). Yet in very psychologically minded centers like the CPC, patients resist precisely such holistic evaluations. Outside of such centers, physicians like Black are in a minority; patients and physically minded clinicians collude in their search for "objective" evidence showing an underlying organic condition causing the pain.[10] Kleinman (1982) considers this collusion to result in a misrepresentation of a much more complex reality (see, for instance, Melzack and Wall 1983:222–231). Many doctors, however, are uncomfortable with the vague language involved in psychiatric explanations of pain, adhering to what Black calls "tunnel vision" (1979:32). And as Kleinman has noted, many physicians find it difficult to talk about interconnections between physiological and psychological causes because of the stigma of mental illness (1982:121).

It is thus understandable that when patients encounter comments from clinicians about pain-proneness (prior mental or emotional factors causing or influencing a pain problem); primary, secondary, or tertiary gain;[11] or possible concurrent psychosocial causes, they are not usually received readily or graciously—regardless of whether these suggestions are made in an indirect, obscure, academic, or excessively blunt manner. Even though a psychologically minded physician may try to reassure the patient that he or she is *not* suggesting that "your pain is imaginary"[12] or "you have a mental problem," the patient will very likely see the physician as suggesting just that. Although both the patient and physician would like to find a physical, objective cause, patient hostility results when one medical procedure after the other is ineffective and the physician finds it increasingly difficult to fit the patient into the customary diagnostic categories. The patient increasingly considers alternative, "illegitimate" diagnoses (see Aronoff 1985:xxiii). Patients feel betrayed by this process, since they depend on the physician for establishing the legitimacy of the pain.

Since chronic pain syndrome patients are "difficult" patients with "intractable" (untreatable) pain, it is no surprise that many physicians prefer to wash their hands of them (Wall, quoted in Benedetti 1974:265). This reluctance is often communicated in some fashion to patients, increasing their uncertainty, suspicion, and hostility and making them even more "difficult."[13]

Table 1 illustrates some of the many ways the notions "real" and "unreal" pain are discussed in the literature. The schematic nature of the table

TABLE I   Commonly Used Clinical Meanings of "Real" and "Unreal" Pain

Real Pain	Organic, physical in origin and maintenance; patient not seen as responsible for pain
Unreal Pain	
Somatized	Psychosomatic (some aura of "real" insofar as there are peripheral inputs, e.g., ulcers). Ultimate cause seen as psychological
	Possibly some "real" pain (e.g., neurotransmitters amplifying pain experience), but main cause is emotional (e.g., pain from depression seen as "real" in the sense of somatized pain, but "unreal" in the sense that if the patient takes care of the depression at least part of the pain will disappear)
	Originally a "real" pain (e.g., car accident) but maintained because of "unreal" reasons
	Primary gain. Can be partly "real" (e.g., herniated disc) but also due to early childhood experiences, "pain proneness," unresolved grief, "caretaker behavior," etc.
	Secondary or tertiary gain. Can be partly "real" but also due to gain from, e.g., being "paid to be in pain" from disability or litigation awards
	"Real" pain, but these physical causes are not the ones patient believes are at work; "unreal" in the sense that patient *is* responsible for cause: not taking care of oneself (lack of exercise), smoking, drinking, obesity, overmedication, substance abuse
Imaginary	Hysterical, hypochondriacal, hallucinatory: no current somatization (although original cause may have been "real," e.g., a car accident)
No Pain After All	Malingering

is misleading insofar as it suggests tidy, mutually exclusive categories, or insofar as it suggests that a given patient fits only one category.

An oversimplified syllogistic schema of the division between real and unreal pain is as follows: (*a*) real pain originates and is maintained by well-understood organic factors whose causes are completely beyond the control of the patient; (*b*) any pain with inputs from psychological factors is to some degree unreal because of the nonphysical nature of these causes and the problematic nature of responsibility for them; (c) the patient has chronic pain in part or in toto because of psychogenic factors; (d) therefore, to the degree the pain is psychosomatic, psychiatric, imaginary, pretended, and so on, the pain is unreal.

This brief account of the perplexing nature of chronic pain syndrome illustrates the thorny problems encountered in the literature and in daily clinical practice on pain units. Because of these problems, patients who enter pain centers are often confused, resentful, and mistrustful. This is extremely important for understanding their discourse about real and unreal pain.

The Pain Unit and the Research

The Commonwealth Pain Center, a separate twenty-one-bed inpatient unit in a private, nonprofit rehabilitation hospital, offers a multidisciplinary, one-month program geared to reducing chronic pain and teaching skills for coping with it. Treatment involves a team approach focusing on conservative, noninvasive therapies, including physical therapy (exercise, whirlpool, ice massage, ultrasound, transcutaneous nerve stimulation); cognitive therapies (relaxation training, biofeedback); social services; group psychotherapy; and one-on-one psychiatric therapy. The main goals of the CPC (and many other pain centers around the country) are eliminating the source of pain when feasible, teaching patients their limitations, improving pain control, relieving drug dependence, and treating underlying depression and insomnia. The CPC also attempts to examine issues of secondary gain, tries to improve family and community support systems, and in general works at returning patients to functional and productive lives.[14]

In the view of CPC staff members, some patients enter the service with an acknowledged-by-all "real" problem with overlays of depression or "pain habits." Others are admitted with what was originally an organic problem (e.g., caused by a car accident), which no longer appears to account for much of the current problem. Other patients come to the unit with mysterious pain problems about which staff has only clues and hunches. To be able to make a more comprehensive diagnosis, staff uses what patients consider prying and provocative tactics. No patients are admitted with "uncomplicated" chronic pain—due to arthritis or osteoporosis, for instance—which they appear to handle reasonably well (see note 7).

The unit was founded in 1972; as of 1984 it had evaluated four thousand chronic pain sufferers, half of whom were admitted as patients. A sample of the patient population from 1984 included 58 percent females and 42 percent males, with an average age of 45.2, and a pain duration of an average of 76.2 months. In 1982, 45 percent of patients received some form of employment compensation. The majority of patients seen at the CPC suffer from lower back pain. Next in frequency are headaches and neck pain, followed by facial, chest, arm, and abdominal pain.[15]

Patients at the CPC follow a highly structured routine. Daily activities begin at 8:00 A.M. and end at 9:30 P.M. or later. Patients' schedules include group and individual physical therapy, relaxation training, psychotherapy, patient community meetings, group excursions to restaurants or movies, group meetings and rounds with the director, group meetings to which family members are invited, conferences with social workers, and meetings with primary nurses. In addition, patients intensively interact with one another in informal groups. Staff insists on attendance at all activities and explicitly encourages patient interaction; at family nights the patient community is told: "It's no secret: you do eighty percent of the work here." Staff also discourages the wrong kind of patient interaction, telling patients to watch out for patients with negative attitudes or patients who want to be taken care of (e.g., have their trays carried, have their beds made). The unit encourages upbeat attitudes and promotes independence and self-sufficiency.

Tough Love and Hard Feelings at the CPC

Perhaps the most striking thing about the CPC is the almost palpable, intense affect in the air. Everyone, including visitors and staff from elsewhere in the hospital, comments on it. The intense affect results in part from the profusion of surprises encountered by newly admitted patients. Some mistakenly expect a fairly orthodox medical facility, others know that psychotherapy is a significant part of the package, and a very few anticipate a more complex rehabilitation for their condition. But all report being genuinely surprised, many extremely so, by the actual situation they encounter.[16] None seem prepared for a program that (1) rehabilitates through independence training, (2) addresses long-standing psychosocial problems that are causing or complicating the pain problem, and (3) weans patients from overdependence on powerful drugs, the medical system, and "pain habits" developed over the years. Thus, most patients experience CPC staff behavior, which is directed toward these goals, in a dazed and muddled fashion. Some patients are confused simply by being told by clinicians in a hospital setting that a goal of the program is to diminish or end their patient careers.

All patients are surprised by the patient community feature and by what I call the "tough love" feature of the program. Tough love ranges from a stony-faced insistence that you continue with physical therapy exercises even though pain is increased, to instances of confrontational therapy, or what I call "paradoxical therapy."[17] Many patients report being baffled by what they perceive as lack of compassion on the part of staff, unprofessionalism, deliberate disregard of the Hippocratic oath, or simple meanness. Patients endlessly discuss their encounters with staff, attempting to explain and reconcile themselves to what they describe as harsh, insensitive, untherapeutic, or simply dumb behavior.

The program's "tough love" therapy has led to a rich lexicon of pithy language about the center: "boot camp," "detention center," "torture chamber, but it's a pain center, so what do you expect?" "concentration camp," "when you graduate from here you deserve a medal," "we're like prisoners," "they treat us like some sort of retards," "they're out to brainwash us," "drill sergeant," "Nurse Ratchet," "this place runs on fear." Yet patients also comment that they understand and approve of the "tough" independence-training approach:

> I thought it was [going to be] like a hospital. But the goal here is to do things for yourself. I think that's good, it's the only way you're going to function.

> No more consoling hand holding. No more of the nurturance that many people were used to getting. And I agree with it. It's either go or no go.[18]

A few patients, some of whom are psychotherapists or clinicians themselves, begin to figure out the "tough love" aspect of the program early on. Others remain confused about it throughout their stay and explain their experiences in terms of individual staff members' personalities. When asked about how intentional and systematic this aspect of the CPC program is, very few patients see it as a conscious policy to the degree it is:

> Some [fellow patients] I've spoken with seem to think it's his [the director's] approach, a consciously practiced technique. To me it's not a strategy, maybe it was before, but now it's unconscious, just his style . . . to have people say things, like "winner," "loser," "here if you succeed, you'll succeed in the outside world."

> I realize the director has to draw a fine line, but at times he's too harsh, it's unnecessary and it's not helped, it's put them deeper into a shell and it takes longer, using this technique—if it's a technique—or just ignorance.

Things are never dull at the CPC: petty or major crises occur daily. Their causes are manifold. Constant pain makes many people emotional, and some patients are being detoxified from narcotics and major tranquilizers. In addition, some patients are undergoing the strain of getting through their first week on the program, a particularly disorienting time. Some have become upset about roommates, the foul language they hear, or any number of other issues. Others are dealing with crises at home, which of course affect their mood. Others are engaged in Wagnerian battles with the director, their psychologist, their individual physical therapist, their primary nurse. And some patients are extremely concerned about how the CPC is evaluating them because of ongoing litigation connected to their pain problem. The CPC's evaluation at discharge can figure prominently in eventual payment settlements, and some patients fear that since staff seems to want to get everyone back to work full-time, they will give an unfavorable (i.e., very low) disability rating (see Jackson, n.d.1).

Thus, while both patients and staff are at the CPC to address the negative consequences of a pain problem, just how this should be approached is the basis for much disagreement. Even those patients who say they are content with their treatment regimen will complain about how other patients are handled. And, perhaps more important, patients disagree among themselves.

PATIENT ENCOUNTERS WITH CPC IDEOLOGY

Encounters between Patients and Staff

Of the many surprises patients encounter at the CPC, some of the most important have to do with the impact of CPC ideology and policy on their notions of real pain. Most patients are all too aware of possible suspicion on the part of others that they may be making more of their pain problem than they need to.[19] They respond to this suspicion with increased resistance and anger, as well as confusion and doubt. Many also say they are demoralized by their unending pain and their many memories of people hinting or saying outright that their problem is not one of "real" pain from a "real" cause, or at least not entirely.

While patients have many grievances about the medical community, they seem to complain most about clinicians' doubting the organic, legitimate nature of their pain problem.[20] Many patients enter the CPC already extremely hostile toward the medical community:

> My opinion of the medical profession has gotten worse. They don't learn. They say, "It's in your head." Doctors should be more humble; if you don't know, say so. A surgeon told me I had to have surgery or I'd be paralyzed later.

> Any doctor who says it's the patient's fault [if the treatment didn't work] should be barred from practice.

Two points should be noted from the last quotation: first, that the doctor is saying that if the problem were "real" the treatment would have worked, and, second, the onus for the treatment's not working is on the patient.

Upon admission to the CPC, patients find that the ultimate authority regarding a pain problem rests with the very same types of clinicians with whom they have had such bitter previous experiences. The vast majority of patients subscribe to a biomedical model of pain cause and treatment, although occasional holistic chiropractors or Native American shamans appear in treatment histories. Patients are in a continuous and difficult dialogue with their memories of encounters with clinicians, with materials they have read (their own medical records, books, and articles), and with one another about their pain problem and its status in the biomedical paradigm. Possible answers as to why their pain is so mysterious, complicated, severe, and unending include the following: (a) this is a medical mystery (the diagnosis may be found in the future), (b) the medical professionals are incompetent and wrong, or (c) chronic pain patients are weak, lazy, or crazy. None of these is satisfactory.

Many patients report being initially put off by the perceived heavily psychological atmosphere of the CPC: "We looked around, we saw psychology there, psychology here, psychiatry there. I got the idea it was going to be a head trip. I felt I was emotionally and mentally sufficient to handle things the way they were." And the vast majority of patients at one time or another disapprove of what they perceived as the staff's position toward their pain:

> I think it's a cop-out to say chronic pain is caused by their mental state.

> There was this notion I was suffering from depression and I just didn't think I was suffering from depression. The treatment, it was like they were justifying their role by forcing you to believe you were depressed.

> They say they *don't* say "depression causes pain," but they do.

> Dr. B in that meeting said all the patients are masochistic. I couldn't believe it, but I heard it.

One enormous area of disagreement stems from patients' understanding of the chain of events that led them to their present state. Many freely admit that they are *now* emotionally disturbed or depressed. But patients will stress that depression or emotional disturbance is the consequence of pain rather than existing prior to the beginning of the problem:

> Mind you, mentally I had lost my mind at that point.

> Because I was so absorbed with pain . . . [I] had lost moments of coherency and I was becoming psychotic with pain.

> I'll tell you something we all agree on: pain causes depression, not vice versa.

Hence, one source of confusion comes from patients saying not that all their problems are entirely "real" but that their emotional problems are a result of the pain: "Fanatics. They totally subscribe to a state-of-mind explanation. When they point out how tense I am I get pissed. Of course I'm tense!"

The staff is elusive with its use of the phrase "real pain."[21] Patients sometimes think that when staff members tell them "all pain is real" this means that they agree that CPC patients' pain is not "all in your head." One patient, a nurse, explained what she thought staff members were saying:

> And I tell them, the community that I speak with, that "your pain is real, the pain came first but what happened psychologically when you're in pain is the depression, is the tension, and it's like being on a merry-go-round and not knowing where to get off. They are so intertwined that you can't separate the two anymore."

But to many patients this model of the intertwining of psyche and soma still implies that their pain is "in their heads"—and caused by depression. Furthermore, staff members contradict this model with many other statements about the ways in which they understand pain to be psychogenic and about how people are responsible for the condition in which they find themselves.

Disagreements between staff and patients about the degree to which patients have a "real" problem arise in discussions about reasonable activities and plans upon discharge from the unit. A patient who was very much in favor of the program nonetheless said:

> They're saying, "Well, if you don't want to work, that's your tough luck, you're able to work." And for insurance purposes they probably have to have something that says, "Yes, the patient is better." Or maybe they believe it . . . I don't know what the rationale is. . . . Maybe it's just so the patients won't leave with a false sense of euphoria. Who knows?[22]

While all patients at the CPC can be said to have chronic pain syndrome, each has a different pain problem and a different history of treatment. Staff determines that some patients upon admission require no medical attention whatsoever, whereas others require diagnostic work or medical procedures. Thus, patients have ample opportunity to see doctors and nurses and other hospital personnel discussing and providing medical services. Resentment and envy about such selective attention to patients' problems often surface. Such differential treatment contributes to individual patients' confusions regarding the status of their own pain problem in terms of "real" or "not real." Thus, while staff will from time to time say that no pain is all psychogenic or all physical, patients tend to see in the lack of attention to diagnosis and orthodox hospital procedures a message that their (or others') pain is all or mostly "in their heads."

The staff directly tell patients that their problem is not as intractable as they perceive it to be, and this, too, contributes to patients' uncertainty about the nature of their condition. When patients are told that their problem can be alleviated via mechanical or cognitive means (e.g., physical therapy exercises can increase circulation and bring relief, or biofeedback can aid in reducing muscle tension), or that their pain can be relieved by adopting a different attitude, doubts and resistance often appear. Some patients voice concerns about whether the staff is wrong in their case and worry that physical therapy will produce further damage. Or they fume that they don't believe in this meditation "mumbo jumbo." Patients are placed in a bind: on the one hand, some hope is being offered for pain relief; on the other, the suggestion is clear that their notions about their pain are wrong. Staff often suggest that the patient has a misunderstanding of what "real," "physical" pain is and what causes it, but staff members are also quite heterogeneous in their own views of what causes pain. (One, for example, gave a lecture and demonstration on reflexology.[23])

As noted, many patients enter the CPC rather wary of the "head stuff" part of the program, especially those who angrily maintain that "here it's all psychology" (meaning the staff is intentionally deceiving them). Yet many patients are simply confused about what the encounter groups and other parts of the CPC's psychological program have to do with their back, neck, or abdominal pain. Patients vary in their views of the psychological program; some heartily approve: "I believe Dr. B's talk about people, [that] their drive, what they choose to do. . . that what would be a total disability in some people is not a disability in others. Not because the level of pain or injury is any different."

A few patients felt the CPC resembles a psych ward—the nurses are psychiatric nurses, and patients learn on their first day in the unit that a psychiatrist and two psychologists are on the staff (the director also holds a degree in psychiatry). However, from time to time the staff affirm that the CPC is a multidisciplinary unit and should not be thought of in purely psychotherapeutic terms. One patient was chided for using overly psychological language: "I was told, 'Don't use words like "termination" with me. Those are psychological terms and this is a medical unit!'"

The Patient Community

Most patients are interested in having their pain seen in organic terms by both staff and fellow patients. This is also a goal of the patient community as a whole in its attempts to publicly construct "real pain" as a shared symbol. This struggle to have "real pain" acknowledged and affirmed affects the formation and functioning of the patient community in two important respects: first, as illustrated above, much of the opposition between staff and patients revolves around this issue; second, this matter profoundly affects the sources of and limitations on patient solidarity.

Initially patients view other patients as like themselves, having a legitimately organic complaint and as sources of support for their own claims to having real pain. One recently arrived patient, discussing why the patient community was so easy to relate to, commented:

> Like on the outside if you hear somebody talking about pain, they're complaining all the time. . . you don't know how much of that is in their head or whatever, or they are just trying to get out of work. Well, here they are not trying to get out of work.

Another neophyte noted: "There's no psychosomatic illnesses here. . . I think everybody here really is in pain, physical pain."[24] Patients comment on feeling accepted by their fellows, with the implication that on the outside talking about pain invites censure:

> It's safe to talk, you're free to talk about pain. . . because it's a real no-no [on the outside] and [here] people will respond and not think you're weird.

> In focus [group therapy] I heard someone pouring out *my* story. I didn't have
> to ask, the things that I wanted to say that were already being said and I'm
> sitting there going, "wow."

Another patient's initial reaction: "You feel a lot less isolated. I'll take that
away with me, because I [now] know that when people complain when I
grimace, it's *their* problem." Many patients commented that being with other
patients helped because they felt as though for the first time their problems
were being taken seriously and that others really believed them: "And after a
while no one believes you. Even my wife."

Patients frequently remarked that the patient community advised and
sometimes pushed them: "Yes, I think there's a sense of trust. You can believe what the other people are saying very quickly." And some patients take
it on themselves to push more recent arrivals because of their experiences
earlier in the unit:

> Last night I gently made somebody to go out to the restaurant. I wondered if
> she was going to feel awful afterwards, but I felt that she could do it because I
> had done it a few weeks earlier and I told her how the first time I went out I
> was a basket case, the next time I was only half a basket case. And she went
> out, and she was a basket case but she was up this morning and said "thanks."

Despite the comments from virtually all patients that the therapeutic community supports and encourages them, patients do not entirely support one
another's struggle to establish that they have "real" pain. The impetus for
much mind- and soul-searching about one's pain problem comes from
input—sometimes rather "tough love" in nature—from fellow patients.
Many patients who initially report feeling accepted and believed by other
patients soon find they must struggle in some way for credibility at the CPC
with *both* patients and staff. One patient we'll call John remarked early in his
stay:

> To be in a place where, when you hurt, you could simply stand up in the
> middle of a conversation and say, "Excuse me," and walk away and go lie
> down and nobody would think that you were weird or feel offended.

But John was also beginning to feel pressure from other patients to sit and
walk rather than lie down: "[but] I am willing to put up with the fact that
sometimes somebody teases me a little harder than I want."

Some patients are quite aware of the role the patient community is expected to play in helping individual patients "get into the program." The
following comment reveals disappointment that the staff is not doing its share
in this regard:

> That's why I'm upset right now that the staff is letting some of the new mem-
> bers be as reclusive as they are. No community member would approve of

someone laying down. If they need to, yes. But if they don't, the staff should run
them out and give us a crack at integrating them into the unit.

Several patients told of being openly recruited by various staff members to
help other patients by not accepting their assessments of their problems and
needs, and by getting "tough":

> Sometimes . . . we were told . . . from the staff . . . for instance, to withhold
> physical help—the trays, mats, and so forth. [Sometimes] I'll listen and then
> stop listening [to patients' complaining about pain], or speak about something
> else. It *is* practiced—trying to remove that behavior.

Indeed, I was struck by the extent to which some of the patients who most
resisted staff definitions of their own problems were such ideal salesmen of
CPC policy to fellow patients. Fred's description of Davie's encouragement is
one such example: "Davie said if I didn't give one hundred percent, the only
one I'd be screwing would be myself. So I started giving all. 'If it helps, fine,
if it doesn't, it doesn't,' I said."[25] Davie was an especially angry migraine
patient whom staff saw as so disruptive that during a special public meeting,
involving both staff and patients, the director told Davie he was being discharged that day. Davie called his lawyer, made an appointment with the
hospital director, and ended up staying on the unit, later being voted in as
vice president of the patient community. Davie resisted much of the CPC's
approach throughout his stay, but many patients told me about how "tough"
Davie was with them and how he encouraged them to "get into the program,
give it one hundred and ten percent."

This approach-avoidance attitude toward CPC ideology on the part of
some patients is perhaps a stage in their coming to accept at least some of the
CPC position on chronic pain. The denial and resistance to what the staff is
telling them, contradicted by what they say to their fellow patients, may
indicate that they are not quite ready to accept their pain as less organic, less
"real" than they thought. However, they *have* come to see some of their fellow
patients' pain as not entirely organic and real.

Clearly most patients experience enormous support and encouragement
from their fellow patients, even though at times this takes the form of
pressure:

> The motivation power of the community is astounding; I guess it's like that of
> these Jim Jones fanatic religious groups in a sense. Ultimately it's being put
> towards a very constructive purpose.

> I look at them and say, if they can do it I can, or if not, there's something wrong
> with my head.

In this last remark, the patient is commenting that if he does not improve,
even with the example of other patients' progress motivating him, *then* there

is something wrong with his head. This is a reversal of the viewpoint most patients hold upon admission.

Almost all patients are surprised at the lines of opposition that can appear between individual patients and staff members and between the patient community as a whole and staff. Some maintain that such structured opposition is inappropriate in a hospital setting: "It's like labor and management, and it shouldn't be." Or they will concur that some conflicts may be necessary but argue that it is overdone at the CPC: "A line has to be drawn, but not a wall built." Some patients perceive patient support and solidarity as a consequence of the difficulties between patients and staff: "Patients. We get emotional support from the patients, not staff. Maybe that's why they're [patients] so active, because of the need to repair, not just from our pain but how to survive here." Some patients speculate about whether the solidarity found in the patient community is intentionally created by the CPC staff and is part of the design of the CPC program:

> I don't know if it's because they [staff] don't understand or it's basically designed that way.

> I don't think it's intentional. I don't think it's planned that the community will try to support each other better because of this. [But] it may help to create patient solidarity.

Many examples illustrate solidarity-building behind the barricades. One patient noted:

> I had the word "manipulative" put on me. I didn't like that. And the only interesting thing about it was that the therapeutic community does grow stronger in reaction to that kind of staff attack. The support from community members who had been saying, "What? You're not a manipulator, you're asking for the right thing."

Clearly the bonds among patients are made stronger by difficult interactions with staff—whether intentional or not. And certainly many of the changes that take place in patients' thinking about pain, particularly about their own pain, come from interactions with other patients. This results from the similarities and differences patients share with one another. Most patients say they feel a sense of camaraderie and empathy with other patients, yet interviews and field notes reveal that patients observe one another with critical attentiveness. This critical attentiveness limits solidarity, at least of an all-accepting kind. Staff members see this as an important component in how the patient community functions as a therapeutic community. Although patients often maintain that "my case is different," many acknowledged somewhat ruefully toward the end of their stay that they had come to recognize similarities between their own previous behaviors and attitudes and those they witnessed in other patients, and that this recognition had been an impetus for change.

CHANGES IN NOTIONS OF REAL PAIN

Some rather spectacular improvements do take place at the CPC: some patients come in on stretchers and leave walking five flights of stairs. Such successes, along with verbal self-reports about improvement, constitute evidence that the CPC is "doing its job." However, patients can and often do resist drawing this conclusion. They may, for example, approve of the physical therapy component of the program while maintaining that the psychotherapy component falls short of the mark. Or they may claim that the CPC is a good program for some kinds of pain but not others. Or they may claim to have tried a "mind-over-matter" approach, but with no success:

> [I was] hearing [that] if my mood was better, possibly the pain would go away. But . . . I *tried* willing it away. I figured, "Well, if I did it to myself, I can get rid of it." And I kept telling myself, "I don't want you, get out of here." Didn't work.

A mixture of optimism and doubt emerges in many patients' assessments of changes in other patients' condition, particularly in their opinions about how long any improvement will last. An excellent example of the complexity of self-reporting is the formal good-bye speech given by each patient about to be discharged. These speeches tend to be upbeat and are often viewed by patients to be somewhat hypocritical, as suggested by patients' commentaries in the solarium[26] after these sessions. One patient, talking about these too-good-to-be-true good-bye speeches, commented: "A lot of people come to the pain clinic [and hear the speeches] and they say, 'I'm not going to say those lies' [but end up saying them after all]." I heard many such comments after formal good-bye speeches. Not only is it impossible to say which version of the CPC's effectiveness was most accurate, but, in my opinion, assuming there is only one true version is simplistic. Up to the day they leave and even after departing, many patients are of two minds, if not more, on the subject of whether the CPC "worked" for them.

It is in discussions of why some patients improve and others do not that patients reveal most strongly their suspicions of their fellow patients. Although some, when asked, "Why do some patients improve and others don't?" answer that to a large extent the differences in improvement are due to differences in original pain problems, the vast majority of interviewees list nonmechanical, nonphysical reasons: personality, socioeconomic position, whether the person chose to come to the CPC, personal history, level of stress, level of emotional problems, "how much you believe in this place," motivation, being ready. One said, "Attitude, attitude. I think almost all pain can be overcome, or managed at least, somehow."[27] While virtually all patients interviewed felt that their own pain problem was basically of physical origin, sooner or later most patients tried out on themselves some of the ideas floating around the CPC, especially those patients at a loss to explain in totally physical, "real" terms why they were feeling better: "My wife calls, 'How are you?' 'Fine.' 'Why?' 'I've been doing lots of things.' 'But that used to make you worse!' It's hard for me to say. It's the community . . . it may distract me."

The biomedical model of pain etiology, which does not espouse that changes in attitude can lead to reduction in pain, places patients in the CPC in a bind. Insofar as treatment is not conventional medical treatment or adjunct treatment that can be explained in biomedical terms (e.g., ice massage brings more blood to the afflicted area), improvement forces patients to admit that to some extent "it's all in your head." Clearly, articulating that one's improvement is due to "motivation" or the "kick in the butt" has far-reaching implications for one's original model of one's pain problem. Such language indicates that patients no longer view their problems as "real" in the sense of a purely organic problem in need of purely medical attention. Undoubtedly this bind is one reason some patients are reluctant to state outright that a change in attitude has actually reduced the amount of pain they experience, even though they themselves have concluded this is the case.

To concede that something like attitude, or even insight, can affect one's pain can be interpreted as "willing" a reduction or elimination of pain. But this can also imply that one willed one's pain into existence, violating the cardinal rule determining legitimacy in Western cultural notions about illness—that one is in no way responsible for one's condition.[28] A clear thread running through many of my discussions with patients is the issue of moral responsibility for their condition: "all-in-your-head" pain implies that to some degree you have brought this problem, involving enormous suffering for you and your family, on yourself. Admitting that one's pain problem is connected to mental or emotional processes invites the stigma of mental illness,[29] or the implication that one is weak or lazy:

> I was aware, but I didn't believe it. And deep down I still don't. I wanted to find a cause, a medical cause. . . . If it was medical, you'd think you were stronger. If there's a medical cause, that makes you feel better because you don't want to accept that you aren't handling things well in your life.

A small minority spoke openly of guilt and shame. A woman with cluster headaches commented that she feels more responsible for "an emotional pain or depression" than she holds people responsible who have pain as the result of a car accident, although she feels her depression resembles the fate that "came ringing against them and took away their self-esteem" in that the effects are so similar.

After some time at the CPC, some patients do openly admit that they had been manipulative in some way:

> They get no sympathy whatsoever in here from staff—and most people are used to, by the time they get in here, some sympathy from the professionals because they've learned how to con the professionals into sympathy. I, for one, was an expert at that, that's one of my major issues that I've worked out since I got here.

Even internally contradictory statements about responsibility reveal anxiety about it: "Whereas I am the opposite, I don't want them feeling sorry for me because it's not their fault, and most of it is not my fault, so why should they feel sorry for me?"

Despite the damage to one's self-image of admitting that one's pain may not be entirely "real," many patients do consider such a possibility. In initial interviews and conversations virtually all patients describe their pain in "real" terms, but many also add that pain is exacerbated by tension, or that stress can bring on a migraine or TMJ (temporomandibular joint pain):

> If you're fighting, you're definitely getting into worse pain. I was always aware of that. The minute I would even raise my voice or get angry, I would get in terrible pain—worse than I was before. And I would say, "Why did I do that?" I could just feel myself tense up all over.

This patient, like many, connects "real" and "unreal" in terms of a core physical pain and contributing psychogenic factors. Another notes: "It came to me all of a sudden that all pain is triggered in the head."[30]

Occasionally in interviews or conversations I felt comfortable enough to push patients to discuss how they saw their own condition in comparison to that of other patients and the degree to which their pain was due to nonorganic, nonphysical problems. A few replied with extremely interesting statements, such as:

> It's like quitting smoking. Why do they continue to smoke? They've heard it's bad, they've read the information.
>
> JJ: But smoking, that's different, isn't it? I used to smoke, I liked a cigarette with coffee, with a drink. But everyone wants to get rid of pain, don't they?
>
> I used to smoke, I didn't like the taste, I didn't like the smell. But I did it. Some people may find the pain pleasurable. They get attention for being in pain. Smoking was pleasurable, but not the taste or smell. The same with pain. I don't know. Some people may find it useful, I don't know why.
>
> JJ: Do you ever wonder this about yourself?
>
> No. But, yes, I have wondered why it took so long to see the connection between pain and tension.

JJ: Why?

It's hard to admit you're in chronic pain. And that it may not go away. You always think it'll go away. You've got to work hard for it to go away, hard.

This interview was carried out midway through the patient's treatment program, and she was beginning to consider accepting at least part of the ideology of the CPC program. Like most other migraine sufferers in the program who perceive a link between emotional factors and their pain, she had always been more open to the CPC stance than patients with other types of pain problems.

The passage quoted above is remarkable in a number of ways. Pain is not defined in any way, nor are its causes discussed. Its maintenance is spoken of in terms of a habit, even an addiction, like smoking, and yet smoking is a consciously chosen behavior, whereas pain is, presumably, an uncontrollable feeling. And yet the patient suggests, in keeping with CPC ideology, that pain is somehow chosen, albeit unconsciously. She responds that she has not wondered about this pain "habit" with reference to herself, but then notes that it took a long time to see the connection between pain and tension. And then she remarks that a complicating factor is denial, a dissociation from pain, a refusal to own it, to accept that "it might not go away"—a frequently heard comment from CPC patients. And finally she introduces the notion of "working hard" to get the pain to go away, presumably similar to working hard to overcome one's smoking habit.

Whether this patient actually subscribes to these opinions or is simply trying them on for size cannot be known. But her comments illustrate much of what is problematic in patients' attempts to make sense of their pain and to figure out a better approach for dealing with it. The reward of a reduction or an end to pain comes with accepting the notion that you control your pain more than you think. However, this quote suggests that for some people, at an unconscious level, the reward *is* pain, because they find it pleasurable. Or, even though it is a negative experience—like the bad taste and smell of smoking—they get rewarded by the attention paid them. Once again the notion is introduced that if you can get rid of pain by controlling it, you got it in the first place through similar mechanisms.

The CPC message about pain is similar to the disease model of alcoholism. Although you are not responsible for getting this disease, now that you know how to control it, you *are* responsible for the consequences if you fail to do so. But experiencing persistent pain is not identical to an alcoholic's experiencing a need to drink. And the notion that "you have not been responsible for your pain until now, but from now on you are" is difficult for patients to grasp, especially given the suggestions made at times that personal history might help explain why pain, even pain initially produced by a car accident, has persisted.[31] For many chronic pain syndrome patients, buying the CPC interpretation of their pain means accepting that they *were* responsible for the appearance of their pain at its onset or later on. The responsibility a patient has for his or her pain also differs from the disease model of alcoholism in that while one is always a "recovering alcoholic," the disease *can* be controlled by not drinking. No standard, clear-cut procedures exist for eliminating the most serious effects of chronic pain, and we have seen that clinicians disagree about to what extent controlling pain behavior versus controlling the experience of pain is the goal of treatment and the measure of its success.

Those patients who leave saying the CPC has been a good experience for them and who have come to subscribe to its ideology about "being responsible for your pain" interpret this notion of responsibility in one of three ways. The first group continues to see their pain problem as "not my fault": they were rear-ended by a Mack truck, which began a downward spiral of pain and associated negative consequences. What has changed in their lives as a result of the CPC experience, they say, is coming to accept responsibility to "get on with my life in spite of the pain." They affirm they are now more able to cope with the pain than they had been because they have come to see such coping as within their power: "Pain controlled me, now I control my pain." When I somewhat mischievously ask, "If you can control your pain, why don't you just get rid of it?" they say they cannot make the pain go away, but they can control the circumstances of the pain experience to a certain extent. Some do say they have learned to reduce their pain through changes in behavior: "I always looked at it from a physical sense: if I felt stronger I would feel better. But it doesn't work that way at all, and trying to do that, I actually felt worse." However, many maintain that their pain has not been reduced at all. Hence, for these individuals, although their notion of "real" pain has not changed in terms of what it implies with regard to the patient's responsibility for causing it, their notion of pain has changed in its implications for functioning and outlook on life.

The second group *has* come to see the pain itself as their responsibility in some way, and these patients say they have come to terms with this. They say they know they must "get on with" their lives:

> [The CPC's approach] seemed mostly psychology. They really pick your brain, they tell you "it's all in your mind," they seem to put more emphasis on your mind. . . . I have a lot of pressure from my father. Coming in here, I felt better. And I realized that outside stresses *can* affect pain.

And those in this group who say their level of pain is the same say that nonetheless their notion of "real" pain has changed.

Finally, unlike the first two groups, whose reported *experience* of pain itself has not changed at all or changed only moderately, a few patients report a radical change in their pain experience. All these patients have necessarily altered their notions of "real" pain, because the CPC does not do medical procedures such as surgery that might account for such a major reduction in pain in conventional biomedical terms. One young man who was admitted reporting severe pain and incapacitation improved dramatically in mobility and reported a major reduction in pain. He reported that his change was due to attitude, that he simply needed to be taught the proper outlook: "I don't know [why my back problem improved remarkably]. Dr. B said it was probably motivation. Other people have shields, I don't . . . because I want to get on with my life." It is interesting that although he thought everyone considered him an unquestioned success and an example others could hope to emulate, several patients sourly commented to me that this young person could not have had all the pain he said he had from his several back operations, because no one can improve so much in a month. And, as we have seen, he could not account for his improvement in physical terms; he was comfortable seeing himself as something of a "miracle."

DISCUSSION

Patient notions about "real" and "unreal" pain which emerge in discussions about their own pain, the CPC program, and the patient community are complex and confused. What are the sources of this confusion, and why do most patients have so much trouble accepting the CPC's interpretation of their pain problem? Patients' elaborations on the basic dichotomy of "real" and "unreal" pain are influenced by their evolving understanding of what the staff at the CPC is telling them about chronic pain, their own improvement (or lack thereof), and their interpretations and legitimations of their pain problem, particularly as compared to other patients.

We have seen that patients in a pain unit such as the CPC are placed in a bind: insofar as treatment is not conventional medical or adjunct treatment that can be explained in biomedical terms, improvement suggests one must agree that "it's all in your head." Saying one's improvement has been due to motivation has far-reaching implications for one's original model of one's pain problem as "real" in the sense of a purely organic problem that needs purely medical attention.

A small part of the confusion found in patient narratives is due to simple misunderstanding of the accepted medical distinctions in vocabulary about pain, such as *psychogenic, somatization, malingering,* and *psychosomatic.*[32] We have seen, however, that the confusion and struggle experienced by patients are not primarily due to semantic ignorance. Of much more importance in understanding their bewilderment are the following contributing factors: stigma, responsibility, the nature of pain (its invisibility, its subjectivity, its

challenge to Western mind/body dualism), patient demoralization from previous encounters with the medical system, and the CPC's unusual treatment
program.

The stigma associated with chronic pain syndrome contributes to patients' resisting the CPC message. To the extent that a pain condition is
chronic, as is the case with other chronic illnesses, it carries more stigma than
acute illnesses (Kleinman 1988). To the extent a pain condition has mysterious origins, it invites stigma more than an illness whose cause is clearly
understood. To the extent that chronic pain is invisible and unmeasurable,
it, like other subjective, nontangible illnesses, is more stigmatized. And to the
extent that the cause of pain is seen as psychological, the sufferer is seen as
weak, lazy, or crazy. Pain straddles the mind/body distinction and thus challenges many of our most deeply held assumptions about biological and mental processes. CPC patients' confusion mirrors most Westerners' perplexity
about processes that connect the mind and body.

Because of these features, chronic pain syndrome can easily baffle any who
might wish to assess responsibility for a given illness. A broken bone may be
seen as "all your fault" because you insisted on going mountain climbing,
but surely this ailment is at the mild end of the fault continuum. It is a sports
injury, visible, mechanical in nature, easily analyzed, and usually easily
cured. At the CPC, the question of responsibility, at times couched in terms
of fault, permeates discussions in far more extensive and puzzling ways than
if broken bones were the topic.

Pain patients' previous experiences with the medical establishment also
contribute to their confusion. Difficult and frustrating encounters have led to
doubts and suspicion, and yet most of the meaning and legitimacy accorded
to their pain problem necessarily comes from the same kinds of clinicians
who elicit patients' suspicions. The CPC staff has the challenging job of
trying to wean patients from overdependence on the medical system, show in
what ways the medical procedures patients underwent were inappropriate,
and yet also affirm and demonstrate how this same system *can* help them.[33]

Finally, despite its claim to espouse policies and procedures contrary to
standard medical treatments, the CPC nonetheless still concerns itself with
discovering which part of a patient's condition is "real." The CPC is called
on to make evaluations and recommendations regarding a patient's status in
civil and criminal suits and in workmen's compensation insurance and other
third-party carrier disability decisions.[34] Most often these decisions rest on
determining to what extent a patients' pain is "real."

If the CPC wants to gain the patient's cooperation, it must convince them
of the advisability of trying a given treatment. This requires patients' accepting the CPC's diagnosis, at least to some extent. And yet the CPC staff
seldom makes clear, straightforward statements about psychogenic pain
because this tends to get patients so angry that they resist therapeutic inter-

ventions. Some patients pack up and leave after a short time in the center; during one period of my research the rate was 33 percent. In general, staff hints and suggests, although no-holds-barred statements will be issued when staff decides to openly and collectively confront a patient. The various deliberately duplicitous, paradoxical interventions (discussion of which cannot be undertaken here because of space limitations) also contribute to a generally confusing situation.

Finally, the fact that the staff represents many disciplines (social work, physical therapy, psychiatry, psychology, neurology, etc.) results in some heterogeneity in staff views about chronic pain. Some staff members are extremely conventional in their medical outlook while others do patient workshops on reflexology and "love medicine" (derived from Siegel 1986).

In short, the sources of confusion for CPC patients are numerous and for the most part cannot be easily remedied by improvements—for instance, in staff-patient communication.

While a comprehensive discussion of the connection between the meaning of pain and patient improvement cannot be given here, I will briefly comment on treatment outcome. While mechanical improvements made by patients during their stay are observable (e.g., range of motion), for the most part indices of improvement take the form of verbal and written reports from patients. Such subjective measures are potentially quite inaccurate, especially if we are concerned about predicting long-term outcome. Evaluating improvement is thus tricky, indeed, and here I will limit myself to pointing out that only a minority of the patients I interviewed before discharge evaluate their own and other patients' condition as *significantly* improved.[35] A minority convert[36] to the CPC's ideology.

I do not mean to imply, however, that the confusion and negative emotions many patients feel during their stay on the unit are correlated directly with failure of the CPC to do its job. Indeed, one purpose of my research was to argue *against* such overly simplistic notions. Following suggestions made by Kleinman (1988:121) and Havens (1986) on paradox, it is possible that the confusion patients experience on the unit is an extremely important ingredient in the shift some of them make in the meaning that pain has for them. An analogy would be the "brainwashing" certain intensive language-teaching methods utilize because of the need to first break down assumptions about language derived from one's native language before being able to introduce the phonology, grammar, and semantic structures of the language to be learned. Insofar as this occurs at the CPC, and I believe it does to some extent, we can see that what appear to be confusing and contradictory statements and policies are in fact instances of a systematic mystification of pain—a feature of the CPC's treatment program.[37] However, since it is also true that institutions reproduce the ideology of the social system they are embedded in, to some extent the confusion about chronic pain in the CPC's program can simply be seen as derived from and reflecting the mystery of pain in the larger society.

NOTES

1. Research at the CPC was funded by NIMH Research Grant MH41787-01 and sabbatical funds from the Massachusetts Institute of Technology. My deepest thanks to the staff and patients at the Commonwealth Pain Center for supporting the study in so many ways. I also wish to thank the following people who gave so generously of their time reading earlier drafts of this paper: Mary-Jo Good, Arthur Kleinman, Paul Brodwin, Byron Good, David Napier, and Rhoda Halperin.

2. In this they match the general profile of chronic pain sufferers who see their problems as organic and needing medical, sometimes surgical, treatments (see Randle 1975:350).

3. See Knoll 1975:367; Menges 1984:1257; Merskey 1978:22.

4. See also Chauvin 1975:353.

5. See Keyes (1985:164), who discusses how the experience of pain is a "shock" in the sense that the sufferer is forced to break with a common-sense perspective on the world.

6. Which the sufferer experiences because of sins committed. Moral responsibility for one's condition is a key feature in any discussion—whether by clinicians or patients—of chronic pain, and one that distinguishes it from acute pain. Acute pain is considered to turn into chronic pain after the somewhat arbitrary cutoff point of six months.

7. Chronic pain syndrome involves pain that takes over a sufferer's life: "If a man has pain from degenerative disk disease but doesn't complain about it, is working full-time, and has a good relationship with his wife, he doesn't need external contingency management" (Schaeffer 1983:24). This is a person with chronic pain but not chronic pain syndrome. Also see the disagreement between Black 1975 and Bonica 1985.

8. Several CPC interviewees volunteered that they would *rather* have cancer than their condition, because it is a known disorder and many types of cancer can be treated.

9. See Pinsky 1975.

10. See Clark's thorough discussion of this search for diagnostic objectivity (1984:114–126).

11. Primary gain "is the intrapersonal, psychological mechanism for the reduction of (defense against) unacceptable affect or conflict. Secondary gain is the interpersonal or environmental advantage supplied by a symptom(s)" (Bokan et al. 1981:331). Tertiary gain involves someone other than the patient seeking or achieving gains from the patient's illness (Bokan et al. 1981).

12. Some doctors do speak of "imaginary" pain in their classifications; see Wingerter's tripartite scheme of real, psychogenic, and imaginary (1975:359).

13. CPC patients always laughed and wisecracked when, during the monthly evening seminar on love and healing, a rehabilitation associate would tell them about

Siegel's argument that it is the "difficult" patient who improves the most (Siegel 1986).

14. From documents on file at the CPC.

15. Information from an internal document at the CPC.

16. Many patients complain about being misled by CPC brochures and intake interviews with respect to the exact nature of the program. Sample comments about these surprises:

> The biggest surprise was that I thought it was a treatment program.... It's not. You aren't treated for pain—not at all.
> I thought it was a way to get rid of that pain. Yes, I got that impression from the brochure.
> I thought it was more of a medical situation, workup and then treatment and rehabilitation.
> And there is really no medicine as I would say being practiced here, I mean there is no heavy staff of surgeons and nurses.
> Not quite as I expected... my family and even myself thought that there was going to be more medical studies.
> [The brochure] was an encouraging, hopeful line. You knew it was PR... I read it as testing—mylograms, thermograms. They didn't talk a lot about the psychological aspects of the therapy.... I'd been expecting the million-dollar workup. Specialists would help me solve the problem.

17. Confrontational therapy is oriented to confronting the patient about maladaptive behaviors; for example, saying, "If you're paid to be in pain [i.e., receiving disability or awards from litigation] you won't improve." Paradoxical therapy is a deliberate attempt to dislodge the patient from a point of view or set of behaviors by disorienting him or her. Both are deceptive to some degree, although paradoxical is more so (see Maranhao 1984). Strictly speaking, paradoxical therapy is practiced in family therapy (see Palazzoli et al. 1978). An example of confrontational therapy:

> The director rejected her excuses for lack of cooperation, insisted on participation in the program, and confronted her superficiality and submissiveness. He prescribed the tricyclic antidepressant doxepin and titrated the dosage upward despite the patient's complaints and anxiety... her attempts at idealizing the therapist were repeatedly interpreted as childlike [from documents on file at the CPC].

18. Since I can discern no correlation between what is said in the quotations given in this chapter and specific attributes of the speaker (e.g., age or sex), I have not included any of this information.

19. And a few are already quite suspicious upon admission, having heard from their families or physicians that pain centers are "for crazy people." Such notions, when communicated, create further confusion in the picture patients have of the place where they are spending a month.

20. Other frequent complaints pertain to iatrogenic complications, malpractice, and policies about medication, most specifically under- or over-prescription of narcotics and tranquilizers.

21. How complicated distinguishing between the two can be is illustrated in the following extended quote from a member of the psychology team:

> There's something very slippery about them [the patients] . . . the psychiatric component
> and the somaticization component, yet they're not totally psychiatric and the problem
> itself is even ambiguous. Nobody ever knows to what degree their pain is real . . . to what
> degree are they beefing it up for secondary gain reasons and to what degree is this person
> really in physical pain—where is it organic, where is it not organic?
> JJ: OK, now "secondary gain": are you talking about conscious beefing it up, or uncon-
> scious?
> Well, there's both, but I think more on the unit would come through as the unconscious
> secondary gain.
> JJ: But there's something about what you just said with the term *real pain*—that uncon-
> scious secondary gain would not be included in your *real pain*?
> Well, I guess when I say *real pain*, what I mean is validatable, or whatever, organic
> reasons for the pain.
> JJ: But, experientially, you're saying that that is real pain for the patient or not?
> I'm using the term loosely; I think that emotional pain is just as real as physical pain.
> JJ: But that is a process so that, even though it is mediated by the central nervous system,
> there is some pain in some part of the body?
> Yes. Once again, they're both connected, you know.

This staff member notes that not only are patients "slippery," with respect to having a foot in the "psychiatric" and "somatization" camps, the problem itself is ambiguous. Although the meaning she is assigning to her terms is not totally apparent, she
is clearly distinguishing between less physical ("psychiatric") and more physical
("somatization") causes and effects. She makes a clear distinction between "real"
physical pain, pain that has validatable, organic causes, and pain that is in some way
not real, pain caused by secondary gain motives, adding that these are unconscious
for the most part in CPC patients. But she then argues that emotional pain can be
"just as real," defending this contradiction with comments about using the term
loosely and about how both types are connected (whether with respect to cause or
experience is not clear). This quotation nicely illustrates the slipperiness not only of
the patients and the problem, but of the term *real* when applied to different kinds of
pain.

  22. And: "I have a feeling that what the staff is saying is, 'You're all better . . . go
back to work forty hours a week.' And that to me is absolute insanity."

  23. Foot massage to relieve pain in other areas of the body. This was a rehabilitation associate on the evening shift; I doubt the director knew about the content of her
presentation, given that he did not believe in acupuncture.

  24. Other examples:

> Some things you can't pinpoint, [but] psychosomatic, whatever, it's real and they don't
> get better.
> It's not emotional. Or psychosomatic, or [an] attention-getting kind of thing.
> And here it's not because everyone isn't trying to get out of pain . . . there's nobody
> pretending that they're in pain here.

  25. This individual, Fred, also a migraine sufferer, had several run-ins with the
director. Fred's account of one encounter illustrates one type of intervention staff
uses:

> I had my first headache the third day. Usually I'd yell and scream and holler my brains
> out. He used reverse psychology and said, "Go ahead, yell your head off, you're only

killing yourself." So I started thinking, who the hell does he think he is? I walked up to him and said, "Do you think that this reverse psychology will work? Well, I'm going to show you you're right and that I'm a better man than you are." So two weeks later he said, "You look like you're doing one hundred percent." I should have had him go down on his knees and kiss my feet.

26. An area de facto off-limits to staff.

27. Other examples:

Those who don't improve haven't gotten into the program.
But yet they walk around cleaning up, making coffee. . . . So, the pain isn't debilitating them, the mind is debilitating them.
Some people can't accept that circumstances in their lives have resulted in a chronic pain condition . . . not being able to express your true feelings.
Well, like, for example, the roommate I had, he left . . . I think he felt he had a lot to lose by getting better 'cause his wife babied him, she did everything for him.
But if you say that to people, their response is to look at you like you're from Mars. Who wants to admit that their life is so fucked that pain is the best part of it?
JJ: But doesn't everyone want to get rid of pain?
I don't think so. I didn't think this before I came in. Some people want to tell people about their pain. . . . He likes it, he thrives on it.

28. Parsons 1951: chap. 10; Young 1980:112.

29. As a staff member bluntly put it, patients resist the notion of psychogenic pain because "it means you're crazy."

30. Another example:

The emotional part of the pain that causes your muscles to tense, and it is intertwined with the pain . . . but a lot of people don't understand it and they really feel that the staff is saying that the pain is not real, that it's in your mind, in your head, it's not a real pain.

31. Staff will point out that, after all, others who have suffered pain from car accidents have managed to get over it, including some staff members themselves.

32. This does not mean to imply that these terms are used consistently in the medical literature. For example, one pain specialist discusses *psychosomatic* in fairly innocuous (with respect to the stigmatizing effects of a link to mental processes) terms: "By this we do not imply the process is imaginary or totally psychogenic, but rather that any disabling physical illness has a major impact on a person's life, family, work situation, and indeed, the patient's total environment" (Aronoff 1982:98). Others take the more generally accepted position of there being some degree of psychogenic cause to the condition.

33. Also, although space has not permitted a comprehensive discussion here, the wide variety of vested interests represented at the CPC, with their distinctive language and agendas, contributes, albeit sometimes only indirectly, to a pain sufferer's confusion. These include: the field of rehabilitation medicine; the subfield of pain specialization; the other specialties that most commonly deal with pain (orthopedics, neurosurgery, neurology); adjunct specialties such as physical therapy; the pharmaceutical industry; the legal profession; the insurance profession. See Sternbach on the doctor having "the role of a double agent, ostensibly working for the patient, but really working for his [the doctor's] sources of income, since the doctor's reports go to every agency that pays his bills" (1978:247).

34. See Corbett 1986 for a fascinating discussion of sessions at a West Coast pain center in which the degree of "real" pain and a patient's entitlement to pain is negotiated among members of the center's treatment team.

35. Using measures concerned with feeling better, being able to do more, and having less pain.

36. What "conversion" means will be comprehensively discussed in a future publication. Here I mean simply enthusiastically accepting and proselytizing about the program.

37. However, I do not mean to imply that this is a conscious policy of the CPC staff. Parallels can be found in the theory behind paradoxical therapy and in various human-potential-movement organizations' policies (see Tipton 1982).

REFERENCES CITED

Agnew, D. C., B. L. Crue, and J. J. Pinsky
  1979   A taxonomy for diagnosis and information storage for patients with chronic pain. *Bulletin of the Los Angeles Neurological Society*, 44, nos. 1, 2, 3, 4.
Aronoff, G. M.
  1982   Pain units provide an effective alternative technique in the management of chronic pain. *Orthopaedic Review*, XI, no. 7 (July): 95–100.
  1985   *Evaluation and treatment of chronic pain.* Baltimore: Urban & Schwarzenberg.
Barrett, R.
  n.d.   Schizophrenia and personhood. To appear in *Person, Self and Illness*, D. Pollack, ed.
Benedetti, G.
  1974   Psychologic and psychiatric aspects of pain. In *Recent advances on pain: Pathophysiology and clinical aspects*, J. J. Bonica et al., eds. Springfield, Ill.: Charles C. Thomas.
Black, R. G.
  1975   The chronic pain syndromes. *Surgical Clinics of North America* 55:999–1011.
  1979   Evaluation of the complaint of pain. *Bulletin of the Los Angeles Neurological Society*, 44, nos. 1, 2, 3, 4: 32–44.
Bokan, J. A., R. K. Ries, and W. J. Katon
  1981   Tertiary gain and chronic pain. *Pain* 10:331–335.
Bonica, J. J.
  1976   Organization and function of a multidisciplinary pain clinic. In *Pain: New perspectives in therapy and research*, M. Weisenberg and B. Turskey, eds., 11–20. New York: Plenum Press.
  1985   Introduction. In *Evaluation and treatment of chronic pain*, G. M. Aronoff, ed. Baltimore: Urban & Schwarzenberg.
Bonica, J. J., and W. E. Fordyce
  1974   Operant conditioning for chronic pain. In *Recent advances on pain: Pathophysiology and clinical aspects*, J. J. Bonica et al., 299–312. Springfield, Ill.: Charles C. Thomas.

Cademenos, S.
  1981   *A phenomenological approach to pain.* Ph.D. diss., Brandeis University, Waltham, Mass.
Chauvin, D.
  1975   Nursing assessment of the patient with pain. In *Pain: Research and treatment*, B. L. Crue, ed. New York: Academic Press.
Clark, J. A.
  1984   *The conversational art of diagnosis: The social construction of medical facts.* Doctoral thesis, University of Colorado, Boulder.
Corbett, K.
  1986   *Adding insult to injury: Cultural dimensions of frustration in the management of chronic back pain.* Ph.D. diss., University of California, Berkeley.
Fordyce, W. E.
  1978   Learning processes in pain. In *The psychology of pain*, R. A. Sternbach, ed., 49–72. New York: Raven Press.
Havens, L.
  1986   *Making contact: Uses of language in psychotherapy.* Cambridge: Harvard University Press.
Hilbert, R. A.
  1984   The acultural dimensions of chronic pain: Flawed reality construction and the problem of meaning. *Social Problems*, vol. 31, no. 4.
Jackson, J.
  n.d.1   Paradoxes, binds and contradictions in chronic pain. Paper given at the 1986 American Anthropological Meetings, Philadelphia.
  n.d.2   Mind and matter: Chronic pain's challenge to subject-object dualism. Paper given at American Ethnological Society meetings in Atlanta, April 1990, in symposium on "The Body as Existential Ground of Culture."
Keyes, C.
  1985   The interpretive basis of depression. In *Culture and depression: Studies in the anthropology and cross-cultural psychiatry of affect and disorder*, A. Kleinman and B. Good, eds., 153–174. Berkeley, Los Angeles, London: University of California Press.
Kleinman, A.
  1982   Neurasthenia and depression: A study of somatization and culture in China. *Culture, Medicine and Psychiatry* 6:117–190.
  1988   *Rethinking psychiatry: From cultural category to personal experience.* New York: Free Press.
Knoll, R.
  1975   Psychoanalysis and pain. In *Pain: Research and treatment*, B. L. Crue, ed., 365–369. New York: Academic Press.
Maranhao, T.
  1984   Family therapy and anthropology. *Culture, Medicine and Psychiatry* 8:255–279.
Melzack, R., and D. P. Wall
  1983   *The challenge of pain.* New York: Basic Books.

Menges, L. J.
1981   Chronic pain patients: Some psychological aspects. In *Persistent pain: Modern methods of treatment*, vol. 3, S. Lipton and J. Miles, eds., 87–98. New York: Academic Press.
1984   Pain: Still an intriguing puzzle. *Social Science and Medicine*, vol. 19, no.12: 1257–1260.
Merskey, H.
1978   Pain and personality. In *The psychology of pain*, R. A. Sternbach, ed., 111–127. New York: Raven Press.
Palazzoli, M. S., et al.
1978   *Paradox and counter paradox*. New York: Jason Aronson.
Parsons, T.
1951   *The social system*, chap. 10. New York: Free Press.
Pilowski, I.
1978   Psychodynamic aspects of the pain experience. In *The psychology of pain*, R. A. Sternbach, ed., 203–217. New York: Raven Press.
Pinsky, J. J.
1975   Psychodynamics and psychotherapy in the treatment of patients with chronic intractable pain. In *Pain: Research and treatment*, B. L. Crue, ed., 383–399. New York: Academic Press.
Randle, W.
1975   The role of the social worker as a change agent in the pain center. In *Pain: Research and treatment*, B. L. Crue, ed., 347–352. New York: Academic Press.
Sarno, J. E.
1976   Chronic back pain and psychic conflict. *Scandinavian Journal of Rehabilitation Medicine* 8:143–153.
Schaeffer, P.
1983   Learning to be a chronic pain patient. *Aches and Pains*, vol. 4, no. 4 (April): 21–25.
Siegel, B.
1986   *Love, medicine and miracles*. New York: Harper & Row.
Sternbach, R.
1978   Clinical aspects of pain. In *The psychology of pain*, R. A. Sternbach, ed., 241–264. New York: Raven Press.
Stone, D.
1979   Diagnosis and the dole: The function of illness in American distributive politics. *Journal of Health Politics, Policy and Law*, vol. 4, no. 3:507–521.
Tipton, S. M.
1982   *Getting saved from the sixties*. Berkeley, Los Angeles, London: University of California Press.
Wingerter, T.
1975   Occupational therapy for the patient with intractable pain. In *Pain: Research and treatment*, B. L. Crue, ed., 359–363. New York: Academic Press.
Young, A.
1980   An anthropological perspective on medical knowledge. *Journal of Medicine and Philosophy*, vol. 5, no. 2:102–116.

CHAPTER SEVEN

Pain and Resistance: The Delegitimation and Relegitimation of Local Worlds

Arthur Kleinman

Chronic pain's uncertain etiology and even more uncertain treatment, its inseparability from the local worlds of sufferers' lived experience, its changing forms and significance in different social contexts, perhaps above all its intractable opposition to interpretation—all make it a particularly rich subject for anthropology. Chronic pain challenges the simplifying Cartesian dichotomies that still are so influential in biomedicine and also in North American culture: for example, the complaints of chronic pain patients regularly defeat easy definition as based upon "objective" or "subjective" evidence. The condition perplexes most those family members, clinicians, and researchers who have not liberated their thinking from "real" (i.e., physical) versus "functional" (i.e., psychological, therefore imaginary) categories.

Bioethicists, who are so preoccupied with the ethnocentric principle of personal autonomy as to regard it as the only solid ground of ethical choices in the hospital, do not know what to make of chronic pain. They do not want to hold cancer patients accountable for their pain; yet the bodies of most other chronic pain patients either reveal no biomedically ascertainable pathology or only such modest pathology that it seems grossly incommensurate with complaints or the cost of care. Are these millions of sufferers responsible for their conditions? Should their care be rationed because it is not "really" necessary? Are they malingerers? Because most workers disabled by chronic pain earn considerably less from disability support than from their job, because many have taken years to grudgingly receive even the limited, stigmatized compensation they do win, and because many are seriously depressed by their disabled condition, it is hard to see one's way to the standard claim of political conservatives that rewards for illness behavior directly encourage malingering (Osterweis et al. 1986). Psychodynamic, behavioral, and most social psychological conceptualizations, though they may at times help in the care of a particular patient or even a special group of patients, also appear seriously inadequate when applied to the broad, multiform class of chronic pain patients.

Social science research on chronic pain syndromes has in the past emphasized the obvious economic costs of these conditions—costs to the healthcare and disability systems and to industry and the economy generally. The professional discourse of economists and political scientists—the latter constructing the terms for political debate over disability compensation—dominate policy analyses of chronic pain (ibid.). Sociologists, who have studied the institutional settings where pain is treated, such as hospitals, clinics, and rehabilitation units, have drawn attention to the negative consequences of the medicalization of pain: professional misuse and abuse of dangerous and expensive tests and treatments, patient experiences of enforced dependency and alienation, and the transformation of human experience into a bureaucratized object and even standardized commodity: *the pain patient*, for whom countless drugs and all sorts of standard and off-beat interventions are marketed as *pain relievers* (Kotarba 1983; Strauss 1970). Studies have repeatedly documented that pain patients feel biomedical practitioners routinely delegitimize the experience of their illness, pressing them to believe that it is not real or, at least, not as serious as they fear it to be (Hilbert 1984). Their subjective reports of distress are challenged, and disconfirmed. They feel violated by practitioners, betrayed by biomedicine. And that enervating and deeply angering sensibility carries over into their family and work settings (Corbett 1986; Kleinman 1988a:56–99).

The questions for anthropologists, then, are perforce diverse. They overlap with the topics that other social scientists have seized upon, yet reflect abiding interests in medical anthropology: the political economy of disability; the social construction of illness categories; the cultural structuring of the course of illness as a form of experience; the biocultural interactions between family, work, and the psychophysiology of the person in pain; the micropolitical use of symptoms as idiom of distress and rhetoric for conducting interpersonal negotiations; the ethnography of therapeutic communities; the differing reactions to care across gender, ethnic, and class lines. The chapters in this volume attest to this diversity of interests, exemplifying how even members of the same anthropological research group construct the subject of anthropological enquiry into chronic pain in rather different ways. Pain's sheer inexhaustibility as a subject for conceptualization and empirical study is a statement about how deeply its roots tap the sources and express the forms of human conditions. Pain eludes the discipline's organized explanatory systems as much as it escapes the diagnostic net of biomedical categories.

Against this background, I choose to address two sides of chronic pain: (1) how, in the context of local moral worlds, different intersubjective experiences of suffering get constructed, and particularly, in the case of pain in North America and China, how that construction turns on experiences of delegitimation and relegitimation; and (2) how one particular cultural interpretation—conceptualizing the experience of chronic pain as the embodiment of *resistance*—can represent the possibilities but also the limitations of anthropological interpretation of suffering.

I will draw on the illness experiences told to me by several of the patients in the Harvard study to illustrate these aspects of chronic pain. Elsewhere (Kleinman 1988*a*), I have written illness narratives of three of the patients I interviewed in order to understand the varieties of suffering as moral experience. Here I sketch the outlines of several exemplary narratives in order to demonstrate how pain emerges in local life worlds as *resistance* to the lived flow of interpersonal experience and in the micropolitics of social relations that have come under larger, menacing societal pressures. To further develop this line of analysis, I draw a comparison with chronic pain patients I interviewed in China (Kleinman 1986).

LOCAL MORAL WORLDS AND THE INTERSUBJECTIVITY OF EXPERIENCE

In his evocative, if enigmatic, thesis on *The Normal and the Pathological* (1989), Georges Canguilhem, the middle link in the intellectual chain of modern French philosophers of science from Gaston Bachelard to Michel Foucault, argued that the central task for a cultural analysis of science is to disclose how a particular scientific practice constructs the object of its enquiry. Canguilhem reasoned that for biomedicine, at best only a partial science, this construction must begin with the determination of the normal from the pathological. In his formulation, this determination had to reflect two conditions: the *norms* that the dominant social group establishes to evaluate and, therefore, control behavior, and also the vital condition of *abnormality* in the biological processes that participate in experience. Thus, for Canguilhem, the question of disease/illness is simultaneously a violation of the *normative* (the moral structure of society) as well as of the *normal* (the enfolding of that sociomoral structure into the body of the individual—its *embodiment*). The dialectical processes mediating the socially normative and the biologically normal are, for Canguilhem, the ontological *and* epistemological grounds for understanding health and disease.

I wish to rephrase this position to bring it into line with an emerging anthropological theory of human suffering, its sources and consequences (Kleinman and Kleinman 1991 in press). What distinguishes the anthropological theory from Canguilhem's approach, and also from that of phenomenologists such as Plessner (1970) and Merleau-Ponty (1962), who have addressed a similar question, and from Bourdieu (1977, 1989), who has explicitly called for a dialectical resolution to opposing subjectivist and objectivist accounts of social reality, is its emphasis on the central importance of the microcontexts of daily life. This anthropological approach to the study of human suffering also lays emphasis on the crucial work of ethnography to describe how microcontexts mediate the relationship between societal and personal processes.[1]

In the ethnographic perspective, those contexts of belief and behavior are *local moral worlds*, where, *inter alia*, the experience of illness is constructed (Kleinman 1980, 1986, 1988*a*). Local moral worlds—be they an East African village (a classical ethnographic context), an inner-city neighborhood in Istanbul, or a social network in North America's universe of plural life settings—are *particular, intersubjective*, and *constitutive* of the lived flow of experience. They are not simply reflections of macro-level socioeconomic and political forces, though they are strongly influenced by such forces. Within local moral worlds, the micro-level politics of social formations and social relationships, in the setting of limited resources and life chances, underwrite processes of contesting and negotiating actions. Yet local worlds are *not* for the most part so greatly fragmented or disorganized as to be lacking distinctive forms or coherence. What unifies divergent statuses and conflicting interests are the symbolic apparatuses of language, aesthetic preference, kinship and religious orientation, rhetoric of emotions, and common-sense reasoning, which, to be sure, derive from societal-level cultural traditions, yet are reworked to varying degrees in local contexts (Cassirer 1957). These symbolic forms work through individual and collective involvement in local social activities to construct the lived flow of experience. Hence, universal types of loss and menace—death, disease, disaffection—are made over into particular forms of bereavement, pain, and other experiences of suffering. For example, in a sensitive ethnography of the Kaluli of New Guinea, Steven Feld (1982) describes the construction of bereavement out of the memory associations of deceased persons with local places, the cosmology with its charter for teleology, the psychophysiological resonance of culturally marked sounds with similarly shaped sentiments.[2] The outcome is a local world of bereavement that is experientially greatly distinctive, yet is not so completely foreign as to lose all resemblance to what is shared in human conditions.

I place emphasis on the moral processes in these local worlds, because it is the construction of what is most at stake for persons and families which assembles from contested preferences and differing priorities a sociosomatic linkage between symbol systems and the body, between ethos and the person, which is responsible for the power of cultural meanings to provide structure for attention, memory, affect, their neurobiological correlates, and ultimately experience.[3] Experience, seen in this structured way, is only in part subjective. The developing child in her cultural context finds herself part of an ongoing flow of intersubjective feelings and meanings; in a sense, she awakens cognitively and affectively within that flow. How to orient herself, what to orient to, her sense of what is most relevant result from the development of moral sensibility to the local world. Ethnic as well as personal identity emerge in this process of entering into and finding a structured place within the lived flow of experience. Social status, gender, and the micropolitical ecology will inflect those identifications, as will personal temperament. We will become ourselves as well as participants in the local world. And this plurality of influence is the basis of the novelty and indeterminacy of experience. But learning to live within and through the vital medium that emerges when symbolic forms interact with psychobiology places our lives squarely in the local flow of things, bound to others and to the moral meanings that define a local world.

And here, where persons encounter *pain*, is where we need to center the study of its sources and consequences. Thus, studying chronic pain patients means that each must be situated in a local world. That world must be described, and the description must include an account of the experience of pain in the wider context of experience in family, workplace, and community. To understand what chronic pain signifies, what its experience is like, ethnographers must work out a background understanding of local knowledge and daily practices concerning the body and the self, and of misfortune, suffering, and aspiration generally. And they must relate this background understanding to episodes of pain, courses of pain, and other aspects of the world of patients and families and practitioners who are responding to the exigency of pain. They must also interpret pain in the trajectory of a unique life course as it is told to them in a narrative of suffering that emerges from their positioned engagement with a person in pain. And therefore they must include in the analytic focus pain as a culturally constituted object for researchers. This agenda, though daunting, should sensitize the researcher to the generative matrix of processes in the local world through which chronic pain is constructed and by means of which, dialectically, chronic pain contributes to the further construction of experience.

RESISTANCE AND ITS MODES

I must narrow the focus of this analysis because of the requirements for a chapter-length treatment of a still-too-large subject. I discuss chronic pain only with regard to how the relationship between pain and moral world is illumined by two rather different aspects of *resistance*, a current interest of many anthropologists that I find both resonant and problematic. I employ the notion of resistance in the widely shared political sense of resistance to authority and in another somewhat special sense that emerges from my own theorizing about suffering.[4]

Resistance as an Existential Process

In the course of the lived flow of experience in local moral worlds, people come up against *resistance* to their life plans and practical actions (Scheler 1971:46). Resources are limited, often desperately so. The mobilization of force is inadequate, insufficient to achieve success in critical negotiations. And, most predictable of all, misfortune strikes. Loved ones die; others fall seriously ill or become incapacitated. Crops or businesses or marriages fail. Aspirations give way, gradually or, following a catastrophe, in a moment. Demoralization becomes desperate and poisons relationships. Loss, fear, menace derail life projects. For many, too many, vicious cycles of deprivation and oppression make misery the routine local condition. For those in the lowest socioeconomic strata, life is brutal. Persons are rendered wretched as a normal, day-to-day condition.

Bearing afflictions of the body, of the spirit, and of the social network and working through their distressing consequences are the shared existential lot of those whose life is lived at the edge of resistance in local worlds.[5] To this dark side of experience we give the name *suffering*, with all its moral and somatic resonances. Suffering, then, is the result of processes of resistance (routinized or catastrophic) to the lived flow of experience. Suffering itself is both an existential universal of human conditions *and* a form of practical and, therefore, novel experience that undergoes great cultural elaboration in distinctive local worlds (Kleinman 1988*a*, 1988*b*).[6]

Resistance to Political Power

In its more usual sense, resistance has the rather different meaning of resisting the imposition of dominating definitions (diagnoses), norms defining how we should behave (prescriptions), and official accounts (records) of what has happened.[7] We resist, in the micropolitical structure of local worlds, oppressive relationships. Such resistance may take the form of active struggle against dominant forces or a more passive form of noncompliance. The historical idea of resistance, such as that of the struggle of subordinate social groups with superordinate ones, conveys images of hidden motives, false compliance, malicious gossip, passive hostility, even sabotage (see Scott 1985:xvi, 290–291), which, I believe, though seemingly greatly distant from the domain of health, can be, with appropriate modifications, applied to less dramatic daily experiences of suffering, including that of chronic pain patients. Most patients with chronic illness, which by definition cannot be cured but must be endured, do not comply entirely with their doctor's prescription. There is little doubt that this "weapon of the weak" may be at times one of the few forms of resistance to medical authority that is feasible, even though it is often self-defeating.

Perhaps a more convincing example comes from bodily forms of expressing political alienation and resistance to the powers of authority. Starting in 1978, I began a series of studies of survivors of China's Cultural Revolution who were suffering from chronic fatigue, weakness, pain, and dizziness (Kleinman 1986). These symptoms were usually diagnosed as neurasthenia, because no satisfactory biological pathology could be discovered. The neurasthenia patients whom I studied were frequently desperate, often depressed, and angry and alienated. Their illness narratives associated their symptoms with the brutal conditions of the Cultural Revolution. Telling their sickness story was a way of venting anguished grievance and hatred over what they perceived as the sociopolitical sources of their misfortune, which otherwise would have been a dangerously unsanctioned behavior. They also were engaged in negotiation with their work units' political leaders to improve work conditions, change jobs, retire, or return home from distant locations to which they had been involuntarily sent. The expression of their symptoms was a rhetoric of complaint aimed at negotiating improvements in life situations that they perceived as hampered or even ruined by political forces beyond their control. In these instances, bodily complaints could be seen as a means of resisting the diffused political control of the Communist state. Unfortunately, more frequently than not, these bodily expressions of disaffection and resistance, of what Scott (1990) so appropriately calls the "hidden transcript," were unavailing and even worsened personal and family problems. Nor were complaints of neurasthenia an effective means of constructing a collective discourse of wretchedness that was critical of the state and that could challenge its policies. Thus, illness as an idiom of distress and noncompliance with health care, in this Chinese instance at least, seemed to point up the limitations and even self-destructive potential of this form of resistance, a point to which I shall return below.

With this discussion as background, I turn to examine both types of resistance among patients with chronic pain in the local moral worlds canvassed in the Harvard chronic pain research projects.[8] My purpose is to see how useful this approach is in deepening our understanding of the experience of chronic pain as human suffering.

THE DELEGITIMATION AND RELEGITIMATION OF EXPERIENCE

Case 1

Stella Hoff is a thirty-one-year-old Ph.D. biochemistry researcher in medicine who has suffered severe pain for four years following a car accident.

> I could be dead or quadriplegic. As it was, I was totally, totally stunned. Shocked. I sat there and shook. At the hospital they diagnosed a concussion, and I had broken a few small bones in my foot. . . . Otherwise, there was nothing else injured. But right away I could feel pain. . . . And that started the whole process. Four years of pain, surgeries, casts, more pain, more tests, more drugs, more surgeries, bad surgical effects, and now this constant pain. . . . And me, us—our lives ruined. All for what?

Dr. Hoff is tall, angular, intense. A woman of few words, clipped accent, she is often bitingly sarcastic about others and herself. Dr. Hoff is elegantly but simply dressed; her movements represent her persona: quick, controlled, assured. In her white laboratory coat, surrounded by her research equipment and assistants, she looks the very epitome of precision and efficacy. A competent and conscientious scientist, she has also something distant, formal, even cold in her bearing. You need to meet her only once to appreciate a fixed expression of tension in her hyperalert eyes and thin, drawn mouth. The intensity of expression seems contentless: it could be fear, it could be hurt, it could be vulnerability. Once you know her story, there is little question what the intensity is about, however. It is her pain—constant, severe, dominating. Dr. Hoff is fighting each moment to remain in control, fighting not to give in, not to scream.

> If I have gotten anything positive out of this terrible experience it is to be more sensitive to the experience of others, especially patients. I don't think doctors have any sense of how to deal with pain patients. . . . I was infuriated by an orthopedist who told me, "Well, it's just pain."

The words she uses to describe her pain are "exhausting, wretched, unbearable, agonizing." Nothing relieves this continuous pain. It is usually a five on a scale of ten in the morning, gets to seven of ten in the late afternoon when she leaves the laboratory, and in the evening is "at least" an eight. When the pain is greatly exacerbated, "it can be a twelve out of ten." The pain is much worse than any pain she experienced before, and is regularly "excruciating." For her pain symptoms and the related problems, Dr. Hoff sees a primary-care physician once every ten days on the average and specialist surgeons and pain experts. She has also consulted psychiatrists and several practitioners of alterative healing systems.

The pain and associated weakness affect most of her activities. It is extremely painful to work in the laboratory, though she does it. It is too painful to do yard work, clean the house, or cook anything involved or elaborate; she cannot play sports; and because of pain she avoids social activities. Pain keeps her in bed for most weekends each month. Over the eighteen months of follow-up interviews, Dr. Hoff's pain waxed and waned. On one occasion she had "very little pain" and reported "it is not interfering with my life very much." On another occasion the pain was "torturing and grueling," though it lasted at this intensity only a few days.

Dr. Hoff has insight into the personal meaning of her pain: "It has been totally devastating to me. Losses and what they have meant to me." She recognizes the pain has made her irritable, fearful, and overly attentive to bodily change.

On formal psychological testing, Dr. Hoff was found to be experiencing considerable anxiety, irritability, and fear. She felt blocked in getting things accomplished, joyless, and she experienced rage, a desire to smash things, and a strong suspiciousness that others treated her badly, could not be trusted, and would take advantage of her if she did not exercise vigilance. Her psychiatric assessment was consistent with recurrent major depressive disorders for the past three years, for which she had received clinical trials of various antidepressants and psychotherapy, which had, in her words, "improved the depression but scarcely affected the pain."

Dr. Hoff's primary-care physician felt frustrated by her care. He estimated seeing her a hundred times or more over the previous four years. He regarded her as a "classical chronic pain syndrome" patient, and noted that her marital life, work, and problematic experiences with the medical system had placed her in a situation of chronic stress, depression, and "self-destructive" anger. He thought there was a strongly psychosomatic component to her pain. He thought of her as one of the most difficult patients he had treated in a very busy practice. He took that to be the reason that led doctors to "drop her." "Let's face it, Arthur," he said, "she is a problem patient. She's just extremely demanding, and she doesn't get better. I feel I need all my skills and then some to stay in the office with her when things are bad. Also being a biological researcher doesn't help."

Other physicians she consulted complained of the same problems. "You know," said one of the pain specialists,

> she is an academic researcher. She knows the language, the medicines. She's read more of the papers on this thing than I have. And she has had so many negative experiences already that she's wary. And then again she has this way of coming across like an intellectual machine rather than a person. I mean she is cold, no emotions, watching you all the time. I find myself trying to avoid treatment interventions that might possibly lead to bad side effects. . . . I mean it just makes the whole thing so much more complicated . . . difficult. When I see her name on my list of patients for that day I feel on edge myself.

Dr. Hoff, in contradistinction, sees herself as the almost silent bearer of a misery only she and her husband know. "I have worked when the pain is a ten," she states emphatically through lips drawn tightly together.

> Pain is too much for physicians to deal with. Most of us can't tolerate listening to people in pain. We want patients who get better, or better yet if they don't they shouldn't complain. Pain patients like me are a sign of the failure of the medical care system, of something terribly wrong at the core.

Dr. Hoff's anger at her professional colleagues is the other side of her anger at the pain and at herself.

> Look what I lost because of it, and where I am now. I get angry with myself, but I can't express it, never could. I get very quiet, others learn to leave me alone—thus, I don't address it. My anger is even too much for Everett [her

husband] to address. I lose confidence that I can control this damn thing, go on
with it, have confidence in the future . . . get better.

Dr. Hoff is a laboratory researcher, an academic who does full-time
medical research, who says she likes her work and is good at it,

> but I have missed so much time because of the pain and the surgery that I still
> have to prove myself. I've lost time. My generation of researchers has moved
> on: they direct their own labs, have their own research program, some have
> tenure. I'm starting all over again. I've lost three or four years. I have to prove
> that I can put in a full research day, complete projects, that I'm like everyone
> else.

She describes lab life as hectic, pressured.

> Previously I brought all my work home with me. It was bad for my family life
> and my own peace of mind. I felt driven, and would continue to work late into
> the night. I felt something tormenting me, driving me on.

Because of the time she has missed, Dr. Hoff has not received the promo-
tion she believes she deserves, and she feels she has also missed out on professional opportunities, getting her name on papers coming out of the lab,
traveling to meetings, and that even her salary has lagged behind.

> It's distressing to be viewed as a risk. I used to be seen as a rising star. . . .
> There is the constant stress of producing, no matter how I feel, to be produc-
> tive, act successful, present myself as healthy. But I'm not healthy; yet I can't
> be honest about how I do feel. Have to pretend. Also, I don't know myself how
> far I can go. . . . I've never had a chance to find out. I've got to be successful in
> this job: there aren't better ones available. And I've got my grant and am
> turning out the papers, "cutting the meat" as we say around here. But it isn't a
> single objective—I need to do the whole thing, to be a steadily productive, day
> in, day out, investigator—no matter how much pain I feel.

Dr. Hoff is presently negotiating a more stable position:

> They still don't have the confidence in me. I ought to be head of my
> laboratory—the current head is someone who started after I did. I taught her
> techniques. I'm a perfectionist in everything I do and always have been. That's
> why it's so hard for me to accept [the effects of the pain]. . . . Even in writing up
> the data it takes me longer. I've got to do it my own way. It's overwhelming to
> do the research, analyze the data, present it, keep publishing, stay up-to-date
> with the literature, do my part in the marriage, in keeping up the house, and
> still be myself. I once thought I could do it all . . . but now I know I can't.

Accomplished in academic studies, Stella Hoff expected success at a high
level. "I had very romantic fantasies of being world famous." The harsh
realization set in and was intensified after the accident.

I recognized for the first time that I wasn't necessarily going to be famous or successful. I had given up writing . . . and in biochemistry I had my doubts. I didn't think I had the toughness to be a great researcher: to do something original and significant. That's why I worked so hard, spent all those hours. I kind of doubted I could "naturally" develop as a researcher. I started out well, but I soon began to have trouble. It is one thing completing a single study and quite another to undertake an entire project. The summer before the accident I began to get very serious doubts. Things were not going well. I began to think of other jobs; something to fall back on. I had driven to job interviews . . . I was chagrined—almost in a trance of unreality. I didn't like the places I visited and couldn't conceive of myself as simply . . . as simply a practicing [technician] . . . . I know it sounds terribly snobby, but I had always thought of myself as a scientist . . . it was a blow to my ego to interview for that job.

Perhaps this illness has prevented or rather delayed a coming to terms with success. So far I have been potential, not actual, success. I think of not succeeding because of the illness . . . but thinking through this condition . . . I'm beginning to wonder whether . . . [it] is not a disguised form of avoiding failure. I don't think I really believe that, but this set of interviews has set off all sorts of associations I haven't made before. I know there are times when stress makes my symptoms worse—lots of times—but then again I can name several very stressful times in the last year or so when my pain did not seem to be affected at all. I know that psychosomatic relations means in some way my mind should be influencing my illness. Strange to say, my experience is almost the reverse. I don't seem to be able through will or feeling or desire to influence my body. In fact my body seems to determine how I feel.

Regarding her family, Dr. Hoff says with a mixture of sadness and bitterness:

Now, they [her family] get pretty angry at me. They simply don't understand what is going on. In fact, my mother can't bear to talk about my illness. She reminds me how much illness she had, and still had five children, worked, got on with her life. My sickness has really affected them.

In the course of many hours of interviews, Stella Hoff went on to tell me about another side of her illness experience, a side she said she had never spoken about with her practitioners.

Do you believe in evil? I mean, we don't use the term in biomedicine, but it does describe experience. Suffering is an evil. I mean suffering that has no meaning, that brings nothing good with it. There is a spiritual side of my pain. That is what I mean by evil. My spirit is hurt, wounded. There is no transcendence. I have found no creativity, no meaning in this . . . this entirely horrible experience. There is no God in it. . . . It shatters all I took for granted and believed in. I came from a religious family, French Protestants. I was taught to put faith in God. All I was taught . . . all my family and personal life . . . has been shattered, taken away. . . .

Dr. Stella Hoff's experience of chronic pain spills over the frame of any single analytic focus. The richly human echoes and protean complexities quite obviously can (and probably should) be analyzed from a number of different perspectives.[9] From the one advanced in this chapter, I note that the catastrophic onset of her misfortune delegitimates a world of experience that she associates with confidence, control, and success. It is a classic suburban, North American upper-middle-class world of academic achievement and promising professional career. Ambition, competition, and competence are personal dispositions structured within a local moral terrain in which progress is regarded as only natural and the actual range of life choices in fact appears almost limitless. (Dr. Hoff came of age in the 1960s and '70s, before the invention of the new tradition of American decline.) In this post–World War II era of great American wealth and empire, the social reality of the "people of plenty" structures the habitus (embodied cognitive and affective structures) of expectation of great success which reaffirms and recreates a social world preoccupied with winning—all components of the American upper-middle-class cycle of self-improvement and self-promotion.

Yet, there is also the hidden fear of "falling from grace," which helps to focus attention on what is culturally most at stake: economic advancement and social mobility, a secularized soteriology (Newman 1989). Not to rise is a threat to social persona and social esteem; it is often experienced by members of the American middle class as a shameful moral weakness. Dr. Hoff, even before her catastrophic accident, had a gnawing uncertainty about whether she would in fact make it in the high-pressured, high-status stakes of science. She had looked into an alternative applied career as a technician, even though it was close to unacceptable to her disposition and the actual values of her local world.

The accident, the injuries, the awful pain, and even the iatrogenic and frustrating medical care turned that world of experience on its head. In this single sense only, hers is like the experience of the multigenerational, inner-city poor, whose intersubjective world is structured by vicious, brutalized cycles of misery, where dispositions of hopelessness and hatefulness recreate and normalize the on-the-ground social reality—though her far greater resources and memory of a very different background augur for a vastly different future. Nonetheless, Stella Hoff does descend into a world of suffering whose bodily and affective processes structure and are structured by painful social relationships in workplace and family setting. She exchanges a world of aspiration for a world of despair, but unlike the truly disadvantaged, she retains the possibility of reemerging. Stella Hoff loses one world to enter another. Her experience of delegitimation is intensified by the responses of practitioners, who contribute to the disconfirming sense that the symptoms are somehow too extreme, too troubling, too difficult to control. There is the suspicion of amplification or exaggeration owing to psychological problems and "stress." This latent, and at times even voiced, accusation challenges the validity of her illness experience and threatens to add the stigma of mental illness or even malingering. To demonstrate the serious burden of her suffering, the desperate desolation, Stella Hoff, like most other chronic pain patients, feels pressed to dramatize her symptoms. Her pain is twelve out of ten. This patently melodramatic device in turn confirms the suspicions of practitioners. The outcome is a poisoned clinical atmosphere in which trust and support—so central to the healing process—are replaced by suspicion, accusation, and ultimately a pervasive, mutually frustrating resentment that makes empathetic care virtually impossible.

The reverberations of this downward spiral include notably Dr. Hoff's literal experience of a spiritual fall from grace.[10] Demoralization as an intersubjective process of suffering shared by patient, family, and practitioners eventually resonates in existential and teleological language. Here the technical rationality and scientific intellectual devices of biomedicine cannot contain the participatory reasoning of the patient who seeks to understand not how but why, not causal mechanism but ultimate meaning, not reason for treatment failure but chance for salvation (see Tambiah 1990:101–110). Thus, Dr. Hoff's story underlines the capacity of suffering as a transpersonal experience to cross the artificial divides between values and practice, religion and medicine which have become so dysfunctional in the American healthcare system. Pain, then, almost becomes an icon of cultural delegitimation of our society's priorities and practices. Perhaps this is why the image chronic pain patients present is viewed as so menacing, why pain patients are cast so often as modern pariahs.

Can we fit the image of resistance into this analysis too? Resistance, in the sense of barrier or opposition to the local flow of lived experience, clearly applies to Stella Hoff's traumatic injury and its desperate consequences. Yet I would argue that the other meaning of resistance—active or passive counterresponse to micropolitical dynamics and the macro-level forces that either intensify or moderate their effect—also can be made to apply. The trajectory of Dr. Hoff's pain, a particularizing *social course* of illness experience that is inimical to the biomedical claim of a *natural course* that unfolds from the disease process itself, spirals around her research work and the pressures of her academic career. Once in place, complaints of pain are readily absorbed into a language of complaint about the enormous pressures and perceived injustices of academic life. Pain is experienced as bridging somatic and social space. To a certain, quite limited extent, embodied pain sanctions opposition to the way the research experience is constructed, which provides an incremental gain in time and autonomy. Yet obviously these "gains" are very little compared to the losses that Dr. Hoff experiences on account of her chronic pain. More impressively, her chronic pain offers Dr. Hoff an occasion to oppose medical practices that routinely disaffirm her experience of complaints as genuine and serious. And taking up an oppositional stance to authority also obviously resonates with her Huguenot heritage and her personality style. She has become, in the eyes of her professional care givers, a "problem patient": a derogatory, even stigmatizing label, that in my experience not infrequently means the patient is making demands that the practitioner will not or cannot meet. In Stella Hoff's case, more than one hundred visits to a primary-care physician over four years may well be so extensive a resort to medical care that few would see her needs as reasonable. But the source of the problem, notwithstanding the claims of her practitioners to the contrary, may well be the system of care and the actual experience of the care they provide. Dr. Hoff is insistent that her pain, including the fullness of her experience, be taken seriously. Her demands confront the inadequacy of the biomedical, including the psychiatric and psychological, approach to chronic pain. The recipient of iatrogenic treatment, she fights back, mobilizing knowledge, and professional and financial resources that most pain patients do not have available. She turns even her spiritual crisis into an assault on the dehumanizing language of a treatment system that addresses neither ethical nor teleological questions. She resists the inappropriate extension of biomedicine's rational technical manipulations into the domain of deeply intimate human experience that calls for compassion and witnessing. And ultimately her suffering challenges simplistic American cultural orientations about youth, health, and freedom.

And yet, as much as the metaphor of resistance reveals of those sides of the chronic pain experience that are often hidden under other social science rhetorics, other aspects of suffering seem obscured or perhaps even distorted by this analytic schema. There is a definite limitation to the applicability of this perspective, and that limitation indicates a more general problem with the anthropology of suffering. Before I examine that problem, however, I will provide a very brief account of another exemplary experience of chronic pain from the Harvard study. After that I will adumbrate, again very briefly, chronic pain patients' experiences from the research I have conducted in China, for the purpose of drawing a cross-cultural comparison.

Case 2

Mary Catherine Mullen is a thirty-year-old married woman from a poor Irish American family in Boston's South End, a bastion of Irish working-class culture, who has suffered from severe "migraine" headaches for five years. Greatly overweight, with a strong family history of headaches and diabetes, Mrs. Mullen fears that her headaches are not getting better, in spite of various medical treatments, and that she will have to endure them for the rest of her life, as has her mother. Her headaches are associated with a depressed and angry mood for which she sees a counselor weekly, and which has transformed her, she holds, into someone quite different from the shy, smiling, self-effacing person she was as a child and adolescent. Mrs. Mullen attributes the onset of her headaches to her husband's alcohol abuse and the subsequent verbal and physical violence he directed at her, which made him, in her words, "a real Jekyll and Hyde."

When the headaches began, Mrs. Mullen was contemplating divorcing her husband. She was desperate to protect herself, and her then five-year-old daughter, from her husband's violence. She also felt trapped by her lifelong diffidence and incapacity to express her needs. Her husband's inability to find or hold good employment meant that they "lived from one paycheck to the next." The feeling of financial insecurity infiltrated other aspects of their life. There were no medical benefits; they were forced to stay in a room in her mother's house, which was undesirable to all, and Mrs. Mullen had to continue to work in a low-level, dead-end job in a local department store which she detested. Finally, she had the terrible apprehension that her husband would end up physically abusing their daughter, just as she had been abused by her own mother.

Her response to this intolerable life situation was a cycle of dysphoria from desolate depression to explosive anger. When depressed, usually at a time her husband was drunk, she became deeply hopeless and virtually immobile—unable to speak out or even act preventively to protect herself or her daughter. When angry, usually when her husband was sober, she would "lose control": scream, throw things, and shout out a litany of wrongs that oppressed her. She even feared that she herself would eventually batter her daughter, thereby copying her own mother, for whom she had come to have an inexhaustible well of anger.

Mary Catherine Mullen was the illegitimate first child of Maggie O'Leary, described by Mary Catherine as an "irresponsible, rebellious" teenager who had run away from a large family of hard-drinking Irish immigrants, and a much older man, who passed through Maggie's life in several intense weeks and then disappeared utterly. Her mother, whom Mary Catherine claims vehemently was "incompetent to care for me," virtually abandoned Mary Catherine, placing her with her own mother, while she wandered in a near alcoholic delirium from man to man. Finally, when Mary Catherine was six, Maggie O'Leary reappeared suddenly without prior notice one evening and immediately demanded her child be returned to her. Despite Mary Catherine's pleas that she remain with her grandmother, whom she had come to regard as her mother, she was forcibly repossessed and immediately entered into her mother's unstable, peripatetic life. She remembers these years of childhood and early adolescence as lacking in all security. She felt unloved and dangerously threatened by her mother's physical abuse. From this time onward, Mary Catherine felt a deep hatred for her mother. At age fifteen she had a sexual affair with an older laborer, which resulted in an abortion, about which she continues to feel guilt. She now believes that she undertook this relationship and dropped out of school in order to break away from her mother and at the same time "to get back at her for all she had done to me." Soon after the abortion, she began to date and quickly married her current husband.

It is an abiding source of shame for Mrs. Mullen that the young couple eventually had to "beg" her mother to permit them to move into her house because of lack of funds to live on their own. At the time she felt trapped in her marriage, her work, and in her mother's home. She watched impotently as her mother took advantage of the situation, treating her like a maid and not providing Mary Catherine and her family with privacy. In spite of her growing anger, she felt incapable of defending herself by talking back to her mother or husband. "If something is on my mind, I can't say it, fear hurting someone's feelings. Can't say no to people."

Over the course of months, Mrs. Mullen descended into despair. She thought of her life as hopeless, and increasingly she felt inadequate and worthless. At one point she thought seriously of suicide. Then the headaches began. So severe were they that she felt compelled to withdraw to her bedroom, where she locked the door, lay on her bed, and remained in the dark until sleep obliterated her pain. Because of her pain, and in spite of the serious financial repercussion and in the face of angry protests from her husband and her mother, Mrs. Mullen quit her job. Within weeks, she determined that the headaches were so severe that she could no longer do housework or cook for her family either. Her husband took over these activities grudgingly, but over time he became more solicitous and helpful. Despite the absence of health insurance, Mrs. Mullen insisted on visiting physicians, including pain experts, who diagnosed migraine, tried her on various treatments, none of which has controlled the pain, and prescribed bed rest and avoidance of "stressful" activities. She further insisted that her husband and mother assume financial responsibility for these medical visits.

As Mrs. Mullen's pain experience deepened, her mother, like her husband, became sympathetic and began to help with the housework. Her husband quit drinking and has not drunk in the subsequent years. Her mother showed her affection, Mary Catherine asserts, "for the first time in my life."

> They treat me the way I have to be treated [because of the headaches]—considerate. If they are not, I'll kill somebody! . . . Everyone stays out of my way when I have a headache and that's what I want them to do.

Although the headaches have continued over the five years, they have slowly begun to diminish in intensity and to become more "tolerable," though at times, particularly when Mrs. Mullen is "under stress," they return to the former level of severity. The depression has lightened, but the sense remains of a deep pool of hate that erupts into angry outbursts. At these times, Mrs. Mullen will "throw up" to her mother accusations about the past. This is the first time in her life, she says, when she has been able to say the things she always had need to say to her mother but couldn't: namely, how she grew up terrified, feeling unloved and greatly vulnerable. When, at the times she is not in pain, she tries to discuss these problems, her mother still turns away from her, "she can't handle it." But during Mrs. Mullen's explosions of rage, her mother is forced to listen.

The analytic language of delegitimation, relegitimation, and resistance in the interpersonal world of experience seems particularly apt in interpreting Mary Catherine Mullen's experience of chronic pain. Of course, the literature on chronic pain contains numerous accounts of the influence of family processes on the onset and course of symptoms. In fact, this is arguably the major causal pattern that behavioral psychologists diagnose and treat (Sternbach 1978; Turk et al. 1983). Psychoanalytically oriented practitioners and family researchers speak of the "gains" of illness and include in that category the explanation that pain and other chronic symptoms can restructure family relations and communication patterns, which clearly has taken place in Mrs. Mullen's household. Yet, the implication is often that either the circumstances are determinative as behavioral operants conditioning individual behavior, out of awareness of the sick person, or that there is a rational calculus by means of which individual decisions are made that reflect a shift in cost/benefit, a kind of malingering (see relevant chapter in Burrows et al. 1987 and also Turk et al. 1983). I find these implications unsatisfactory and am disturbed by the behaviorist language that would have us believe that Mrs. Mullen is either an ingenuous automaton or a blatant manipulator. Ten hours of interviews with Mrs. Mullen, corroborated by research and clinical work with many patients with chronic pain, make me greatly suspicious of the behaviorist discourse, which I find stereotyped, overly focused on pain as a problem of an *individual*, and dehumanizing.

In the perspective I have advanced in this essay, Mary Catherine Mullen is born into a delegitimated world. Illegitimate, abandoned by her mother, and raised by her grandmother in a family setting where she was viewed as tainted by her mother's sinful ways, Mary Catherine's early socialization disaffirmed her person and placed her in an anomalous relationship with her grandmother and others. She bore a sense of shame and also carried the idea that she was not good enough to receive her mother's love. When her mother precipitously removed her from her grandmother's home, she experienced a major loss and second transformation of her world. That transformation again encouraged an experience of delegitimation. Her mother abused her emotionally and physically. She also forced Mary Catherine to accept the name of the man to whom her mother was then married. For a while Mary Catherine had two family names: her mother's and her stepfather's. The confusion in identity was a simulacrum of her growing sense of tangentiality to her local world. In that world, she repeatedly heard her mother excoriate her origin and personality. Disaffirmed and disaffected, she grew into adolescence feeling worthless. She felt a lack of efficacy with others and alienated from her family.

A common idiom of distress was her mother's headache. When her mother had headaches, which were frequent, Mary Catherine was expected to take care of the other children and her stepfather. Her mother's withdrawal and lack of affection were justified by the headaches, as were her irascible disposition and angry outbursts. Thus, Mary Catherine experienced headaches as a rhetoric of complaint for expressing hostility and controlling others.

The experience of delegitimation was reproduced in her relationship, in the early part of the marriage, with her husband. She seemed unable to control his drunken behavior and its violent consequences. She also seemed unable to effectively negotiate with him over their limited resources, much of which supported his alcohol abuse. After the birth of their daughter, she felt more intensely still the disaffirmation of her experience as wife and mother. Forced to move into her own mother's home, owing to her husband's failure as a provider, it appeared to her that she had come full circle to complete a lifelong cycle of despair. Mary Catherine's great obesity, about which she felt helpless and ashamed, became a bodily index of her alienated social status, a habitus structured out of the conflagration of stigmatized position, poor self-esteem, and a self-defeating sense of inefficacy in her local world. This alienation of habitus in turn structures the negative dispositions and interactions that perpetuate that world.

The experience of pain in a world without security (in family, job, finances, or neighborhood) is what distinguishes chronic pain among the poor and the oppressed. When one cannot marshal resources, symbolic and instrumental, because they do not exist or one's access to them is obstructed, the very idea of control becomes untenable. The normal, everyday routinization of misery, furthermore, can be experienced as bodily pain. As a result, the confluence of this source of pain and bodily pathology makes it impossible for the afflicted person to determine what "causes" pain to worsen and what will limit or remove it. Pain cannot be made meaningful any more than can the rest of life. The absence of control as well as legitimacy means that to survive, those patients who lack resources yet are exposed to great pressures must conduct the moral equivalent of a life-and-death struggle. Pain, in such a local world, becomes the bodily component of so fundamental an experience of suffering that the local world becomes a world of suffering. Pushed up against the limits of control and meaning making, poor and oppressed patients may take up whatever is at hand to respond to adversity that can no longer be easily assigned to either medical or nonmedical sources. Thus, Mrs. Mullen's pain itself becomes a kind of solution, albeit compromised, to the consequences of suffering in her world.

The development of chronic pain, whatever its sources, sanctions a transformation in her experience. The pain becomes a means of resisting her husband's irresponsibility and her mother's cruel manipulations. Her sense that her world is not her own, that she has no central, secure place in it, is replaced by illness behavior through which Mrs. Mullen, with surprising energy and efficacy, moves to the center of that world and even comes to dominate its flow. The severe migraine headaches authorize a relegitimation of intersubjective experience. They are in fact emblems of a new way of engaging in the felt flow of experience. Mary Catherine Mullen's episodes of headache might even be thought of as a kind of social dissociation, from a hesitant, marginal orientation to her world, in which she is absorbed into the flow of practical actions effected by others, toward an assertive, central orientation, from which she reorients the flow of aggrieved sentiments and practices. The relegitimation of the world authorizes her access to the moral devices of accusation and restitution.[11] Of course, there is also evidence that Mrs. Mullen's resistance has certain negative effects, real and potential, such as expensive medical bills, unemployment, and perpetuation of a cycle of somatized distress and greatly disruptive explosions of rage into which her daughter may become the next conscript. Also, it is unclear how long such a newly invented ritual of behavioral reversal can keep going without straining the social ethos to the point of breakdown. For these reasons, it is difficult to know, at this point, if Mrs. Mullen's form of resistance in the politics of family and workaday world should be regarded as effective. What is more certain is that for poor working people from deprived backgrounds with few life chances and greatly limited resources, who lack reserves to respond to crises, even the dubious efficacy of embodied resistance may mean the difference between enduring and succumbing. In the exigency of routinized hurt and grievance and demoralization, simply not to continue to be overwhelmed may be a kind of desperate victory. Pain, like other forms of suffering, is resisted (Scott 1990).

Case 3

An even clearer example of the possibilities and limits of the moral efficacy and practical experiential uses of resistance via chronic illness is provided by the research I have conducted in China among those deeply affected by the Cultural Revolution (Kleinman 1986; Kleinman and Kleinman 1991 in press). In this research, my colleagues and I encountered such frequent examples of neurasthenia symptoms sanctioning major changes in work and family and in relationship to the local Communist authority structure, we concluded that chronic, disabling bodily complaints were a chief source of power in Chinese work units. But it was also obvious that social categories of individuals—those with bad or good class backgrounds, women, youths who had been Red Guards—strongly influenced who had need for such power and who could exercise it under particular conditions. Moreover, delegitimation meant something very different in the Chinese context. Our research subjects, like tens of millions of their Chinese compatriots, experienced the moral delegitimation of communism in the fiery chaos of the Cultural Revolution. Their local worlds, and the societal political system of which these are part, had lost moral legitimacy, and even the sources of social efficacy were undergoing dramatic change. Relegitimation has failed at the macrosocial level in China, both through the brutal repression of the democracy movement and in the failure of the Chinese Communist party to reform. Yet, at the regional and local levels, various kinds of relegitimation efforts have occurred, with varying degrees of success. Hence, in Guangdong and Fujian provinces the economic reforms have continued virtually unchanged, whereas in other, poorer, more violated provinces a Communist counterreformation is underway. Most notably, in many work units and villages, there is a unified opposition to central and regional directives, and informing on others and collaborating with the entrenched political leaders are much less prevalent than during the Cultural Revolution. This is even the case, it seems, within the Communist party itself. In this sense, delegitimation of local moral authority is so pervasive that China can be said to be in the final stage of a cultural delegitimation crisis, even though it is uncertain what will follow.[12] Yet what is certain is that resistance through somatic symptoms and disability has not been an effective means for either expressing collective resistance or ushering in new forms in the local moral order. Even on the personal level it has been more self-defeating and socially unavailing than effective in reconstructing the flow of experience.[13]

For example, a middle-aged teacher in a rural town in Hunan had withdrawn into reclusive existence, mourning her losses in the political devastation of the whirlwind; under the authorization of her neurasthenic complaints, her withdrawal had no effect on the local political situation, but in fact worsened her family problems and deepened her own feeling of desolation. Another neurasthenic patient, a very competent Hunanese school administrator, carried her neurasthenic depression and pain as publicly recognized scars of her personal losses in the Cultural Revolution. Because of her complaints, she had been engaged in negotiations with the leaders of her work unit to either take early retirement or have removed an old cadre who blocked her administrative reforms. Yet her symptoms only made her situation more desperate and did not alter the political impasse in the work unit. A third sufferer of headaches, Huang Zhenyi, experienced a deeply humiliating personal trauma early in the Cultural Revolution, when as a young adolescent he was unjustly convicted of criticizing Chairman Mao. He had become obsessed with the bitterness of the injustice and was trapped in a self-defeating cycle of wishing to right a wrong on behalf of his "lost generation" while at the same time protecting himself from the machinery of political repression. The result was a corrosive political silence replaced by louder and louder physical complaints that deepened his alienation. (These and other stories of Chinese survivors of the Cultural Revolution who suffered from neurasthenia are described at greater length in Kleinman 1986:105–142.)

THE LIMITS OF RESISTANCE AS AN ANTHROPOLOGICAL INTERPRETATION OF SUFFERING

Perhaps I have not done as full justice to the model of resistance as it deserves. Because the research I conducted in Boston involved the elicitation of personal and family narratives of pain and did not include participant observation, my access to local worlds of pain was constrained. This is an important constraint for an interpretation of the intersubjective flow of experience, inasmuch as I have had to assemble that interpretation from personal accounts and brief home visits with family members. In spite of this methodological restriction, I do feel this chapter contains evidence of the utility of the analytic framework in the anthropological study of the social course of chronic illness. Its chief value is as an operational device, which, as I have tried to illustrate, can facilitate analyses of the local mediation between microsocial psychological processes and the macrosociopolitical context. Parry and Bloch (1989:1–32) contend that the short-term cycle of transactions that individuals undergo parallels the long-term cycle of transactions at the societal level: together they *reproduce* cultural forms and social structures. In the perspective that I am advancing, the connection between these short- and long-term cycles occurs within the medium of a local world that situates person and family in an intersubjective space where moral order, affective ties, and bodily processes are integrated into a form of experience that has particular and shared features. The model of resistance, and the closely related concepts of delegitimation and relegitimation of moral worlds, offers only one perspective on this psychocultural mediation.[14] Yet, the limitation of this model, I believe, can be generalized to other anthropological approaches to the study of human suffering.

I characterize that limitation in the following terms. Just as anthropological accounts, such as those in this collection, fault biomedicine for its failure to respond to the teleological requirements of suffering—those existential and spiritual questions of what is most at stake in human experience that query the ultimate purpose of living—so, too, do culturalist accounts, which are so effective in diagnosing the inadequacy of natural science renditions of human conditions, fall prey to a type of social scientific transmogrification of suffering. Thus, interpreting chronic pain as resistance, or for that matter as discourse, gives primacy to the search for meaning over the rest of experience. The interpretive requirements of suffering for theodicy—namely, the struggle of rebuilding a coherent account of why misery should exist in the world (see Weber 1978:518–529)—are viewed by many anthropologists as the core reality of suffering. But, as Veena Das (in press) demonstrates in the tragedy-filled lives of Indian survivors of the Hindu-Sikh ethnic conflict and the Bhopal disaster, most of those who encounter deep suffering experience a chaotic, aleatory world. The wrenching process of having to bear the awful consequences of loss, menace, and the brutality of everyday deprivation are experienced not as theodicy but as terror and desolation and, for all too many, as the abulia of alienation. Whatever its particular features, the inter-subjective experience of suffering is so various, so multileveled, so open to original inventions that interpreting it solely as an existential quest for mean-ing, or as disguised popular critique of dominant ideology, notwithstanding all the moral resonance of those foci, is inadequate. It may distort and even-tually transmogrify this most deeply human of experiences.

For an ethnography of experience, the challenge is to describe the proces-sual elaboration of the undergoing, the enduring, the bearing of pain (or loss or other tribulation) in the vital flow of intersubjective engagements in a particular local world. The ethnographer needs to fasten onto the overriding practical relevance of experience for those who engage in it, for whom some-thing crucial is almost always at stake. At the same time, the ethnographer must struggle not to dehumanize the felt flow of lived experience through professional deconstructions that are totalistic and thereby claim an absolute, unpositioned knowledge of determinants and effects. Such an interpreta-tion must be invalid because it denies the uncertainty and indeterminacy and sheer novelty of human engagements. Experience is emergent, not pre-formed. It changes. It goes on and on. The ethnographer must be cautious about creating an end that is artificial, an illusion of a finality that is not to be found in intersubjective space, where the echoes of embodied memories re-verberate even after a death. The cultural constructionist's icon can be as inhumanely artifactual a characterization of experience, then, as is the pathologist's histological slide.

Properly deployed, the model of resistance must avoid these misuses and abuses of anthropological interpretation. That means that it probably can never be entirely satisfying as an explanatory account of human suffering. And perhaps that is as it should be. For when pain is configured as suffering, it evokes intractable, inexhaustible moral and spiritual questions that are worth pursuing to the extent we can better understand human conditions or provide assistance to sufferers, but which are as vulnerable to dehumanizing social scientific accounts as to biomedical ones. And here anthropologists of pain find themselves in an ethical position roughly similar to that of the clinician. For both, it is essential first to do no harm. For both, the moral requirement of engaging people who suffer is to struggle to transcend limited and limiting explanatory models so as to witness, to affirm, their humanity.

For both, there may come a time when, like the grieving author of the ancient *Lamentations over the Destruction of Sumer and Ur* (Mintz 1984:22), they need to admit, "There are no words!" It is in this spirit that I adumbrate resistance, delegitimation, and relegitimation of local worlds as *figures* to bring forward aspects out of the complex, collective *grounds* of chronic pain that have heretofore been obscured. This is yet another side of a subject that is best dealt with, not by insisting on a single "objective" interpretation, but by juxtaposing multiple, positioned, intersubjective perspectives.

NOTES

1. A considerable body of writing touches on aspects of this anthropological focus on the grounding of meaning and experience in local cultural worlds; see, for example, Abu-Lughod 1986; Geertz 1987; B. Good this volume; Hallowell 1967; Rosaldo 1980; Shweder and LeVine 1984; Stigler et al. 1990; Wikan 1980, 1989.

2. Schieffelin (1976), writing on the same ceremony among Kaluli but from a different theoretical perspective, has also presented a sensitive ethnographic description of this particular cultural construction of bereavement.

3. In this paragraph, I follow Bourdieu's (1989) usage of the terms *structure* and *structural* and *structuring*, but I will hereafter freely substitute the words *construction*, *constructed* and *constructing*, and *constitutive*, within the same general conceptualization of the generative dialectic in social processes.

4. The latter usage of resistance is expanded in Kleinman and Kleinman 1991 in press; the former usage builds on Scott (1976, 1985, 1990), who in turn appropriated the concept from an earlier, largely Marxist, generation of theoreticians, whom he also criticized; the idea of political resistance has been taken up in ethnographic works in which suffering and healing figure by Comaroff (1985); Ong (1987); Martin (1987); Taussig (1981) among others. Scott (1985) emphasizes peasant resistance in class struggles with wealthy villagers; his focus is on the everyday routines and extraordinary actions of participants in local moral worlds, who, among other things, engage in the politics of reputation and the implicit threat of violence to defend their vulnerable positions. Particularly pertinent is his argument that political economic decisions that mandate planned development undermine the established routines in local communities, so that the very moral structure itself is threatened, including the established patterns of interaction across classes. This places the poor at great risk and also threatens their legitimated coping devices. The analogy can be transferred to the health field to emphasize both the structural vulnerability of subordinate groups to local social changes that result from political economic change which in turn place greater pressure on the health status of the poor, and also as a means of highlighting, albeit provocatively, the increasing gap between the technological power and cognitive control of health professionals and the threat of increasing powerlessness felt by patients from the lowest socioeconomic stratum. Under these conditions, the patient-doctor relationship can become such an unequal engagement that poor patients find noncompliance one of their only ways of resisting paternalistic authority and asserting what little personal efficacy they believe to be available to them. The consequence, as Scott (1985, 1990) shows for the agricultural domain and political order

generally, may be to worsen their material conditions, yet the intention is to resist authority and to struggle for more control, symbolic and pragmatic. The same processes of resistance, I contend, occur in the therapeutic relationship and affect the moral economy of health. The political imagery will seem exaggerated and even inappropriate to many health-care providers and planners. Yet I would suggest that for at least some patients of poverty and perhaps for many others with chronic illness, the feeling that they are deploying "weapons of the weak" in unequal engagements both with the practical realities of health care and with those symbolic apparatuses that support society's "tryanny of health" which hold them responsible for their misfortune is neither irrational nor without its uses, particularly if the partisan language of class warfare is replaced by the experiential terminology of the ethnography of suffering.

5. For a useful discussion of embodiment of distress and disease from a phenomenological perspective, see Csordas 1990, whose discussion can be read as a complement to this operational description of suffering.

6. In the Jewish tradition, as Mintz (1984) discloses in his remarkable survey of responses to catastrophe in Hebrew language literature, writers have been torn by two questions that are highly relevant to the issues explored in this chapter. First, how should the suffering of the collective be portrayed? (Ever since *Lamentations* the device has been personification via the experience of particular individuals.) And second, how should unexplained and undeserved suffering be dealt with? The emphasis has been on cognitive disorientation and subsequent restoration of the paradigm of meaning (Mintz 1984:21). This meaning dominated concern with suffering, which has been so fateful for the Western tradition, periodically gave way, especially after the pogroms and the Holocaust, to a concern with resistance, as in Bialik's poem of rebuke of passive acceptance of oppression by Russian Jews following a pogrom, "In the City of Slaughter":

> For since they have met pain with resignation
> And have made peace with shame,
> What shall avail thy consolation?
> They are too wretched to evoke thy scorn.
> (Mintz 1984:140)

The implication is that resistance is both authorized by undeserved suffering and the only morally justifiable response. Thus, the idea of resistance is charged with special moral significance in the Western tradition, a significance that echoes in Marx and in the writings of anthropologists who have picked up this question. This Western orientation toward suffering, especially as it has been refracted in the writings of existential authors, has, on self-reflection, clearly influenced my own contributions: first toward a meaning-centered medical anthropology, and more recently toward an anthropology of experience.

7. See Aaron Cicourel's tripartite model as described in Bourdieu (1989).

8. To protect the anonymity of the research subjects whose stories of pain I elicited, through five to ten hours of interviewing of each subject, I have changed identifying details and provided each subject with a pseudonym. The information contained in this chapter, though altered for this purpose, accurately conveys the essence of the research I conducted. When I have made changes to protect anonymity of patients and practitioners, I have drawn on findings from the entire group of the

chronic pain patients I interviewed in order to insure that the changes held general validity.

9. A full treatment needs to consider each of these aspects of pain. By focusing narrowly, I neither discount these other interpretations nor do I seek to contribute to a fallacy of misplaced concreteness. Resistance and delegitimation are components of a complex, contradictory, only incompletely understandable, positioned picture. I draw them out because others have paid insufficient attention to these moral sides of pain, and they support the larger conception of suffering I seek to develop.

10. I cannot here go further into the place of this religious implication of a fall from divine grace in the Hoff family's Huguenot tradition of Protestantism in Catholic France, but it is worth remembering that besides apostasy and forced uprooting, the spirit of resistance remained a strong component of the Huguenot's ethnic identity. Dr. Hoff's family took their religious tradition as serious business, and Hoff's building of her own career lends itself quite easily to the Weberian interpretation of the Calvinist roots of secular success. Hence, it would also seem appropriate to follow Weber further in his analysis of suffering as *resentment*, a critique of cultural authority from those below the established hierarchy or from those who, having fallen out of grace, take on a pariah status for which they seek retribution (Weber 1978:518–602). Furthermore, as Philip Hallie's (1979) study of how the French Huguenot village of Le Chambon saved Jews from the Nazis and their Vichy collaborators discloses, this tradition of Protestantism has supported political resistance of a remarkable quality, a tradition that Dr. Hoff's family prized.

11. In research with patients suffering from chronic fatigue syndrome in Boston, my colleague Norma Ware and I have noted that their exhaustion, once defined and sanctioned as a medical illness, though it frequently seems to be the result of exhausting life-styles, can also authorize basic shifts in the pace and control over activities in their local worlds. Some of these sick persons, most of whom are women, once they are diagnosed as chronic fatigue patients, make such fundamental decisions as changing or giving up jobs and intimate relationships, and end up transforming the very structure of their lives and even such daily social rhythms as when and how they sleep, eat, exercise, and spend their time. Illness, then, relegitimates their flow of experience and reorganizes their engagements and transactions, authorizing greater control. Michel de Certeau (1984:43) avers that "everyday practices depend on a vast ensemble which is difficult to delimit but which we may originally designate as an ensemble of procedures." Our chronic fatigue patients, at least some of them, altered the "ensemble of procedures" and thereby everyday practices, too, through the experience of illness. I believe this can happen in chronic illness generally, including chronic pain.

12. The phases of this delegitimation crisis are several. During the Great Famine, from 1959 to 1961, when at least fifteen million Chinese and perhaps as many as twice that number died of starvation, hunger reached most Chinese families, yet the press dissimulated bountiful harvests, thus removing the possibility for effective public criticism that might support a challenge to the moral legitimacy of Communist party rule. The depredations of various antirightist campaigns and the chaos of the Cultural Revolution led to widespread private condemnation of Communist ideology and authority. This condemnation was such that in the period of economic reforms, from 1979 onward, the party itself switched its ideological justification for Communist rule

from the erstwhile class warfare to the new claim that communism had improved and would continue to improve the lives of most people, though it was admitted that 10 percent of the population still lived in abject poverty. This ideological reform was an attempt to shift the grounds for moral legitimacy to rule—what the Chinese have traditionally called the Mandate of Heaven—at a stage when massive cynicism had seeped into virtually every corner of the state. The Tiananmen massacre completed the delegitimation of the moral order. Mainland China today is ruled through military power alone without any vestige of cultural legitimacy. For the citizen in his family circle, delegitimation moved from passionate affirmation of Marxism to bitterly enervating disillusionment, and onward to involuntary compliance with discredited authority. Cynicism followed misplaced loyalty. Foot-dragging, false compliance, and passive hostility followed passionately prodigal political fervor and revolutionary ardor. The embodied effects of this trauma are deep and pervasive. (See Thurston 1987; Liang and Shapiro 1983; Cheng 1986; Liu 1990 among others.)

13. Perhaps the clearest North American example of pain as resistance to political authority that I came across in the chronic pain sample was a middle-aged lawyer from a suburban town who had arthritis in his hips and knees. Emile Sachar represented local working-class clients in negotiations with developers and the town authorities in a local dispute. Once his adversaries had recognized that Mr. Sachar's chronic condition worsened over the course of the day and required that he periodically get up, walk around, and even lie down, they pressed for meetings that lasted longer and longer, at which Mr. Sachar found himself sitting in chairs that lacked proper support. He felt certain that the behavior of his adversaries was aimed at worsening his complaints so that he would more readily agree to a compromise that favored their interests over that of his clients. Mr. Sachar responded by deliberately using his disability to authorize official delays in the negotiations. He also pointedly emphasized his pain and its effects on his posture and gait to gain a more sympathetic hearing for his clients' position and even to project the image that they were victims. The downside of this oppositional response, besides its limited tactical success, was the undermining effect the illness behavior had on Emile Sachar's personal life, including his marriage. Indeed, Mr. Sachar's demoralization seemed to arise as much from the social intensification of his disabled role as from his increasing despair over the possibilities for social justice in American society. Thus, like the Chinese patients whose neurasthenia had become the embodied scar of the Cultural Revolution, the bodily mode of resistance seemed to deepen personal crisis while not succeeding as a form of political protest or change.

14. For an alternative analysis of the cultural mediation of experience, see Jackson (1989:1–18).

REFERENCES CITED

Abu-Lughod, L.
   1986   *Veiled sentiments: Honor and poetry in a bedouin society.* Berkeley, Los Angeles, London: University of California Press.

Bourdieu, P.
1977   *Outline of a theory of practice*. New York: Cambridge University Press.
[1972]
1989   Social space and symbolic power. *Sociological Theory* 7(1): 14–24.

Burrows, G., et al., eds.
1987   *Handbook for the management of chronic pain*. New York: Academic Press.

Canguilhem, G.
1989   *The normal and the pathological*. New York: Zone Press.
[1966]

Cassirer, E.
1957   *The philosophy of symbolic forms*, vols. 1–3. New Haven, Conn.: Yale University Press.

Cheng, N.
1986   *Life and death in Shanghai*. New York: Grove Press.

Comaroff, J.
1985   *Body of power, spirit of resistance: The culture and history of a South African people*. Chicago: University of Chicago Press.

Corbett, K. K.
1986   Adding insult to injury: Cultural dimensions of frustration in the management of chronic back pain. Ph.D. diss., joint doctoral program in medical anthropology, University of California, Berkeley and San Francisco.

Csordas, T.
1990   Embodiment as a paradigm for anthropology. *Ethos* 18(1): 5–47.

Das, V.
In Press Moral orientations to suffering: Legitimation, power and healing. In *Health and social change*, L. C. Chen et al., eds.

de Certeau, M.
1984   *The practice of everyday life*. Berkeley, Los Angeles, London: University of California Press.

Feld, S.
1982   *Sound and sentiment: Birds, weeping, politics and song in Kaluli expression*. Philadelphia: University of Pennsylvania Press.

Geertz, C.
1987   *Local knowledge*. New York: Basic Books.

Hallie, P.
1979   *Lest innocent blood be shed*. New York: Harper & Row.

Hallowell, A. I.
1967   *Culture and experience*. Philadelphia: University of Pennsylvania Press.
[1955]

Hilbert, R. A.
1984   The acultural dimension of chronic pain: Flawed reality construction and the problem of measuring. *Social Problems* 31(4): 365–378.

Jackson, M.
1989   *Paths toward a clearing: Radical empiricism and ethnographic inquiry*. Bloomington: Indiana University Press.

Kleinman, A.
 1980   *Patients and healers in the context of culture.* Berkeley, Los Angeles, London: University of California Press.
 1985   Somatization. In *Culture and depression,* A. Kleinman and B. Good, eds. Berkeley, Los Angeles, London: University of California Press.
 1986   *Social origins of distress and disease: depression, neurasthenia, and pain in modern China.* New Haven, Conn.: Yale University Press.
 1988*a*   *The illness narratives: Suffering, healing and the human condition.* New York: Basic Books.
 1988*b*   *Rethinking psychiatry: From cultural category to personal experience.* New York: Free Press.
Kleinman, A., and J. Kleinman
 In Press Suffering and its professional transformations: Toward an ethnography of experience. Paper presented at the First Conference on Psychological Anthropology, San Diego, 7 October 1989. *Culture, Medicine and Psychiatry.*
Kotarba, J.
 1983   *Chronic pain: Its social dimensions.* Beverly Hills, Calif.: Sage Publications.
Liang, H., and J. Shapiro
 1983   *Son of the revolution.* New York: Alfred A. Knopf.
Liu, B. Y.
 1990   *A higher kind of loyalty.* New York: Pantheon.
Martin, E.
 1987   *The woman in the body.* Boston: Beacon Press.
Merleau-Ponty, M.
 1962   *Phenomenology of perception.* London: Routledge & Kegan Paul.
Mintz, A.
 1984   *Hurban: Response to catastrophe in Hebrew literature.* New York: Columbia University Press.
Newman, K.
 1989   *Falling from grace: Downward social mobility in the American middle class.* New York: Random House.
Ong, A.
 1987   *Spirits of resistance and capitalist discipline: Factory women in Malaysia.* Albany, N. Y.: SUNY Press.
Osterweis, M., et al., eds.
 1986   *Pain and disability.* Washington, D.C.: National Academy Press.
Parry, J., and M. Bloch
 1989   Introduction. In *Money and the morality of exchange.* J. Parry and M. Bloch, eds. New York: Cambridge University Press.
Plessner, H.
 1970   *Laughing and crying: A study of the limits of human behavior.* Evanston, Ill.: Northwestern University Press.
Plough, A. L.
 1981   Medical technology and the crisis of experience. *Social Science and Medicine* 15F:89–101.

Rosaldo, M.
1980   *Knowledge and power: Ilongot notions of self and social life.* Cambridge: Cambridge University Press.

Scheler, M.
1971   *Man's place in nature.* Translated by H. Meyerhoff. New York: Noonday
[1928]   Press.

Schieffelin, E.
1976   *The sorrow of the lonely and the burning of the dancers.* New York: St. Martin's Press.

Scott, J. C.
1976   *The moral economy of the peasant: Subsistence and rebellion in Southeast Asia.* New Haven, Conn.: Yale University Press.
1985   *Weapons of the weak: Everyday forms of peasant resistance.* New Haven, Conn.: Yale University Press.
1990   *Domination and the arts of resistance: Hidden transcripts.* New Haven, Conn.: Yale University Press.

Shweder, R., and R. LeVine, eds.
1984   *Culture theory.* New York: Cambridge University Press.

Sternbach, R., ed.
1978   *The psychology of pain.* New York: Raven Press.

Stigler, J. W., et al., eds.
1990   *Cultural psychology.* Cambridge: Cambridge University Press.

Strauss, A., ed.
1970   *Where medicine fails.* New York: Transaction.

Tambiah, S.
1990   *Magic, science, religion and the scope of rationality.* New York: Cambridge University Press.

Taussig, M.
1980   *The devil and commodity fetishism in South America.* Chapel Hill: University of North Carolina Press.

Thurston, A. F.
1987   *Enemies of the people: The ordeal of the intellectuals in China's Great Cultural Revolution.* New York: Alfred A. Knoff.

Turk, D. C., et al.
1983   *Pain and behavioral medicine: A cognitive-behavioral perspective.* New York: Guilford Press.

Weber, M.
1978   Theodicy, salvation and rebirth. In *Economy and society*, vol. 1, G. Roth
[1922]   and C. Wettich, eds., 518–529. Berkeley, Los Angeles, London: University of California Press.

Wikan, U.
1980   *Life among the poor in Cairo.* London: Tavistock Publications.
1989   Illness from fright or soul loss: A North Balinese culture-bound syndrome? *Culture, Medicine and Psychiatry* 13(1): 25–50.

Epilogue

*Mary-Jo DelVecchio Good, Byron J. Good, Arthur Kleinman,
Paul E. Brodwin*

All the contributors to this book conducted their formative field research in societies and cultures outside North America—in China and Taiwan (Kleinman); Iran and Turkey (Good and Good); Colombia, Guatemala, and Mexico (Jackson); Haiti and Senegal (Brodwin); and Mexico (Garro). Each author brings these cross-cultural and comparative experiences to his or her work in American society, and each casts the analyses of the experience of chronic pain for individual patients in terms of contradictions and struggles in particular local worlds of American culture. These conflicts emerge out of the ambiguity of "body" and "mind," "soma" and "psyche," as opposing symbolic domains; the uncertainty of distinctions between "subjective" and "objective" experience; the disputed definitions of reality in professional and lay discourses; the quest for culturally acceptable forms to express the veracity of pain; and the individualizing of experience and responsibility within the context of the family and the professional health-care system. Chronic pain subverts dominant symbolic oppositions in American culture, bringing pain sufferers into conflict with professionals and with medical practices that instantiate these cultural categories. The result is a corrosive challenge to the legitimacy of the suffering of those with chronic pain. The case studies presented here explore this orienting dilemma through analysis of symbolic forms and everyday practices in the lives of individual sufferers and in the local contexts of American medicine.

The research developed at Harvard and presented in this book has its origins in Kleinman's studies of somatization and depression in China. In his monograph *Social Origins of Distress and Disease: Depression, Neurasthenia, and Pain in Modern China* (1986), Kleinman examined the role of "neurasthenia"—a category in Chinese professional and popular culture—in mediating local power relations, social inequities and oppression, and the extraordinary social and political events of the Cultural Revolution and its aftermath. This research was conducted in a setting very different from contemporary North America. "Body," "mind," and therefore symptoms are figured quite differently in Chinese medicine and in popular and literate culture. Chronic pain, though experienced by many neurasthenia patients, received little attention per se from care givers. It was so unmarked that neither the popular culture nor the professional medical nosology possessed a category for chronic pain. At the time of that research, Chinese psychiatry was in ferment. The legitimacy of neurasthenia as a professional category for comprehending and treating dysphoria, bodily pain, fatigue, and weakness was in question. Because Chinese were for a brief moment permitted to publicly recall their suffering during the Cultural Revolution, the political significance of bodily experience became a significant theme.

Kleinman concluded his study by calling for systematic comparative studies of pain and depression. He recommended that studies focus on the ways macrosocial processes work through local contexts to structure the body's relationship to society and our interpretations of that relationship. Specifically, he argued that "we know very little about cross-cultural differences and similarities in the way the body is experienced." He called for "phenomenologies of bodily modes of experience" that would allow investigation of how the body mediates social forces and transacts cultural meanings (1986:191). Kleinman urged special attention to the role of local cultural categories in disclosing "how the self is *created* as a locally shaped experience" (1986:196). The studies of chronic pain in American culture were developed to contribute to this comparative enterprise. They represent a stepping back into our own culture from the culture of others.

A central conclusion to the studies presented in this book is the extent to which the *experience* of the chronic pain sufferer is resistant to incorporation into biomedical and psychological theorizing and care, as well as to ethnographic reporting and social science analysis. In general, the experience of a patient has limited validity within medicine, unless it maps neatly onto the body as source of disease and site of the medical project. Chronic pain resists such mapping. Individuals as well as support groups for pain sufferers are thus constantly involved in a quest for legitimacy. But human experience also eludes social science analysis. Much of the medical social science literature reproduces regnant medical distinctions, although it locates pain's origins in psychological—or social or cultural—processes rather than the body. Little wonder pain sufferers feel their condition is poorly represented in either standard medical description or the language of the social sciences.

Chronic pain comes to meaning in the context of conflicted social relations and contested interpretations: there is no ethnographic stance outside the "politics of interpretation." Anthropologists cannot speak for those in pain. However, anthropology's special message in this field is that the personal

and intersubjective experience of individuals in pain must be given legitimacy and placed at the center of analysis. Cultural meanings, social relations,
and history are all inscribed in experience, and these should be the subject of
anthropological attention. But experience surpasses that inscription. Anthropologists need to return to the centrality of experience—its form and
consequences—in comparative studies of pain.

As we conclude this volume, we point briefly to four questions provoked
by the chapters of this book which should occupy anthropologists and other
social scientists interested in the study of chronic illness and the body's relationship to society. These questions reflect our conviction that new approaches are required for the study of experience. Experience provides a
window on broader social and civilizational processes. At the same time,
experience can be studied only in the context of the narratives through which
it is figured, the broader social formations in which experience is embedded,
and the larger civilizational processes and their relation to local social
worlds.

*1. How can we more adequately represent experience and situate it in our analysis of
chronic pain?*

Experience resists symbolization and therefore often eludes anthropological analysis. Though troubling to the anthropologist and philosopher,
the gap between experience and objectification offers little problem in everyday life. Most of us get on with the practical exigencies of our lives without
consternation or paralysis over the fact that our felt experience of dread or
distress or even pain cannot be measured directly, and therefore cannot be
authenticated. For those with chronic pain, however, as the studies in this
book illustrate, this resistance to recording or representation is a source of
added suffering. In American medicine, attention to the *experience* of pain
often marks it as subjective and therefore beyond objective diagnosis or treatment. Legitimacy and its benefits are withheld, even as treatment seems unavailing.

But the location of pain across dominant medical oppositions is now well
established in the social science literature. Some have even argued that the
analytic observation of pain's ambiguity *contributes* to its lack of legitimacy
(Hilbert 1984). And pain treatment centers such as that studied by Jackson
(this volume) have made pain's subversion of the dominant dichotomies the
source of specialized "paradoxical treatments." The ethnographic representation of the pain experience, therefore, rather than the recognition of the
ambiguous status of that experience in medicine or in social life more generally, remains deeply challenging.

The chapters in this book suggest several directions for the analysis of
experience. The phenomenological tradition provides a rich source for the
study of experience and the perceptual organization of the life world; how-

ever, this literature has invoked such a self-referencing analytic terminology and has paid so little attention to culture that few of its most important technical analyses have been drawn into anthropology. Several anthropologists with an interest in the body and "embodiment" have recently turned to a careful reading of phenomenology as the basis for ethnographic writing (Csordas 1990; see Corin 1990; Jackson 1989). B. Good's chapter in this book analyzes the role of pain in distorting or unmaking the life world of the sufferer and narrativization as a response to the threatened dissolution, drawing explicitly on analytic categories of Alfred Schutz. M. Good's chapter, analyzing life stories of two professional women, demonstrates that work may be another means of remaking the life world, as well as a domain for working through personal sources of suffering drawn into the pain experience and articulated in a conjoined idiom.

Brodwin's chapter, on the other hand, argues for the importance of "performance" as a metaphor for the analysis of experience, elaborating the role of social practices in evoking and representing experience. Illness complaints have an important rhetorical dimension: they are meant to arouse a response in audiences, as well as express discomfort. Moreover, cultural and personal meanings do not exist only as abstract concepts: they are largely enacted or constituted in practices that both express and shape lived experience. Practice, in turn, is constrained by power relations, especially as expressed through institutional and social authorities. Therefore, the experience of chronic pain is organized as much by social constraints and demands for enactments as by solitary subjective awareness. The term *performance*, however, comes with its own ambiguities. Through its association with drama and acting, it carries connotations of the pain sufferer as actor and of pain as having voluntary aspects, a view strongly rejected by many in our studies who described pain as seeming to have its own agency and volition. Kleinman's chapter explores a similar ambiguity in recent writing on "resistance." Kleinman combines a phenomenological account of the origins of the pain experience in the resistance of the body with a critical account of the sufferer as actively resisting oppressive social forces. Although in the end he questions the utility of "resistance" as a metaphor for analyzing the pain experience in China and the United States, his chapter along with Brodwin's suggest directions for representing agency in relation to pain.

2. What is the relation between the experience of chronic pain and the narratives told by pain sufferers and medical professionals?

Anthropologists—along with physicians, family members, and friends of the pain sufferer—often infer the nature of the pain experience from stories told to us by those in pain. Conventional wisdom has it that stories reproduce experience; they represent an account of experience from the perspective of the sufferer. Recent literary critical studies indicate how much more complex is the relation of story and experience. Many literary critics have held that stories are largely cultural conventions, remaking experience in its narrative representation. Others have argued that experience shares with stories a fundamentally narrative quality (e.g., Carr 1986; Ricoeur 1984); stories thus both represent past experiences and provide a frame for organizing our experiences as lived. Along with reader response theorists, who suggest the importance of the analogy of the reader of a text in investigating how we construct experience by seeking to "emplot" it (e.g., Iser 1978), these writers provide the basis for a renewed examination of the relation of stories and experience. Recent writings in psychology (Sarbin 1986; Bruner 1990), sociology (Mishler 1986), and anthropology (Kleinman 1988; Mattingly 1989; B. Good 1990) indicate the "narrative turn" in the humanities and social sciences has the potential to offer new insights into the nature of illness experience.

The analyses in this book drew largely upon life narratives of pain sufferers and stories they told us about experiences with pain and with care providers. To some extent, all the chapters represent reflections on the relation of narrative and experience. Garro's chapter examines explicitly the structure of care-seeking narratives. She demonstrates how individuals reconstruct past experiences in light of emerging understandings, reshaping their life stories in face of the "ontological assault" of pain. B. Good's chapter describes the maintenance of multiple stories by a pain sufferer, when neither a story of pain as resulting from childhood trauma nor a story of pain as a consequence of a joint disorder has the potency to evoke a cure. To date we know rather little about the nature of stories of pain experience across cultures and thus how such stories reflect and evoke experience. The chapters in this book suggest the importance of pursuing this line of research.

3. How is the chronic pain experience embedded in the broader relations of the body and society? How can we undertake a critical phenomenology of the chronic pain experience?

Richard Bernstein (1976:135–169) some years ago argued that phenomenologists such as Alfred Schutz have often shunned "critical evaluation of the different forms of social and political reality"; he argued that a "thorough-going phenomenological analysis" that examines how ideology "systematically *mis-takes* what is relative to a specific historical context for a permanent feature of the human condition" has the potential to make a special contribution to critical studies (p. 168). The chapters in this book have argued that even though the experience of pain is created in or generated by the body, it is also constituted in the body's relationships to society and its local worlds. In particular, the social contradictions present in medical ideologies and their response to pain, in gendered social relationships, and in class and power relations give shape to the modes and dynamics of the pain experience for many sufferers. A study of the experience of chronic pain thus begs for a critical phenomenology.

The chapters in this book examine in various ways how the contradictions of medical theories and practices, as well as reimbursement policies, have profound influence on the experiences of chronic pain sufferers. Chronic pain is marginal to the dominant theories of biomedicine. Pain clinics, along with alternative therapies for pain, have evolved in the margins of medical institutions. In standard medical settings, the bodily and experiential order of chronic pain is framed by ideologies and practices that divide the sufferer into parts and reorder the "pain patient" by practice specialty and clinic schedules. The medical pain specialties juxtapose that which is objective and observable—"image-able" through contemporary technologies, organic, measurable, and testable—to that which is subjective and "merely" told— functional and recalcitrant to measurement, opaque to observation. Outside of standard practice, the treatment of chronic pain is moved into a liminal zone of diverse institutions, pain centers, therapies, and ideologies. Chronic pain patients thus find themselves rejected by standard medical practice and referred to institutional settings that are then vilified as nonscientific, alternative, nonorthodox, and for which reimbursement is unavailable or only marginally legitimate and standards for competent medical practice ill-defined. The resistance of the body to the treatment of pain is thereby amplified in experience by the contradictions of the American health-care system. Thus, the medical institutions within which the experience of pain is interpreted and manipulated, so as to legitimize certain features while the unified whole is delegitimized, define one crucial dimension of the body's relation to society. Over time, through the routines of medical practice, fragmentation is etched into the everyday experience of the pain sufferer (see Kaufman 1988).

Kleinman's analysis of the political dimension of the relationship of body to society in his studies in China suggest further directions for analysis in American culture as well, in respect to hierarchies of power. State politics and state trauma were not factors in the lives of the patients interviewed; if the studies had focused primarily on powerless, poor, and unemployed Americans the picture would have been different. Yet with the exception of Jackson's project, the vast majority of those recruited to these studies were women, working women. The predominance of women, which reflects the clinical epidemiology of chronic pain, suggests that experience of pain and the body's relationship to society are gendered. How it is gendered is as yet problematic, and the chapters in this volume take different approaches to exploring the relationship of women's bodily experiences to society's hierarchies of power. For example, studies have repeatedly shown that in American society, work for women across social classes affirms women's sense of self and competence. M. Good's chapter illustrates that in contrast to popular work stress models, work for professional women who are in positions of power may provide a haven from pain rather than amplify its experience. In addition, the women's narratives in many of the chapters suggest that gender, patienthood, and chronic pain interact to compound the experience of disaffirmation in encounters with the medical profession. Future explorations might examine the way in which interpersonal, family, and community history may be inscribed into the body (Pandolfi 1990), bringing about an experience of pain that is not only *individual* but that also resonates with and represents the events of one's social community.

4. How is the experience of chronic pain configured in the relation between civilizations and local social worlds?

We have referred throughout this book to some elements of biomedical culture and more generally to European and North American civilizational themes that structure theorizing and practices concerned with chronic pain in our society today. In particular, we have addressed how dominant symbolic oppositions, which are part of Western philosophical heritage, play a direct role in marginalizing chronic pain. Our observations are limited, however, and comparative studies will be required to indicate the most important dimensions for comparison (see Brihaye, Loew, and Pia 1987 for a collection of brief sketches of the interpretation of pain in a variety of major religious and cultural traditions). We indicated in the Introduction the importance of a civilization's framing of human suffering and its dominant soteriological convictions. We have suggested implicit comparisons between cultural forms and political relations in China and the United States, and Kleinman's chapter makes that comparison explicit. However, the contextualizing of pain studies in broader civilizational research is hardly begun. We can only conclude with a statement of conviction of the importance of joining ethnographic studies, undertaken in specified local settings, to broader historical and civilizational studies, if we are to understand the role of social and cultural processes in structuring the pain experience. The chapters in this book are intended as a contribution toward this larger effort.

In this regard, we will attempt to summarize a few of the insights the anthropological study of chronic pain warrants about continuities and changes in American society. Nearly all the chapters depict the process of disaffirmation that pain patients undergo as they seek care. The contributors have emphasized the institutional sources of delegitimation. Yet this process is not confined to biomedicine; the pain sufferer experiences disaffirmation in much of social life. What is it about American society that conduces to professional and popular behaviors that routinely question—accuse may be more apt—whether a person's suffering is valid or not? The research reported here suggests several answers.

A number of our subjects complained of something akin to a North American *tyranny of health*. The dominant images in the popular culture extol physical vitality and deny anything short of robust health. Blemishes, illnesses that cannot be rapidly cured, and especially grave infirmities that suggest disability or death are banished from everyday life. A strong will, we are told, can influence the body, so infirmity is often associated with a lack of individual strength (see M. Good et al. 1990). The chronically ill feel great discomfit in this ethos. They are discredited as burdensome, anomalous, and, in some unspoken but definite way, responsible for their condition. Suffering is accorded no positive value. To bear distress and pain is not the same thing in the post-Reagan era as it was in Colonial, Jacksonian, or Victorian America. It now carries no moral virtue. Quite the contrary, in the society of instant crises and quick remedies, of risk management for the unexpected, the very idea of *chronicity*, of predictable, serious, long-term trouble, is unacceptable. Thus, the chronically ill—especially those with conditions that are at the borderline of respectability—feel that they are culturally illegitimate, unaccepted in the wider society.

Quackery has had a long run in North America. From vendors of secret Indian remedies to religious hucksters, from a thousand-and-one kinds of psychotherapy to claims of strange cancer cures, within and without the healing profession, entrepreneurs of therapy have sold the public the latest nostrums and the oldest anodynes. In comparative cross-cultural perspective, the flourishing of folk healing and popular culture health commercialism, even in a highly industrialized society, is unexceptional. Yet it runs counter to the rational technical models that dominate public health and health policy. Chronic pain highlights the kaleidoscope of healers and healing practices. It is not simply that biomedical misadventures drive those with chronic pain away from the established therapeutic systems. Rather, the relative inefficacy of standard biomedical approaches has opened a space for entrepreneurs to compete for market share. The unstable boundaries between science and commercialism and between medicine and religion, as well as rational technical models that configure economic costs but not suffering, are standard features of America on the brink of the new millennium. Chronic pain seeps through the porous barriers between the different sections of society. The sociologists' standard map of American social structure looks woefully outdated when matched against the institutions traversed by pain patients. A study of the difference between how institutions define their own activities and how they actually operate in this country could have no better subject matter than the quest for the relief of pain.

Medical anthropology has in recent years sponsored an increasing number of studies in North America. Yet compared to studies of health and health care in non-Western societies, studies initiated in North America seem to have made less of a contribution to understanding the cultural and social dynamics of the wider society. While the narrow technical orientation of many studies may be at fault, there are other reasons that suggest a more formidable problem. The immensity of American civilization, with its plural life worlds and rapidly changing crises, creates grave uncertainty about how to generalize from any single field study and determine which issues are primary and which derivative. American culture's extreme emphasis on individuality also contributes to the problem. The researcher is always challenged to justify generalizations projected onto the collective, when individual and local differences abound and heterogeneity can be found throughout the cultural *and* political and economic systems. We believe the failure of anthropological studies to effectively move beyond health and medicine to American culture per se results in part from these constraints. And we have to admit these constraints are visible in our own chapters. Nonetheless, in looking ahead toward the decade of the 1990s, it is our collective view that medical anthropology in American settings must contribute more substantially to American studies.

Finally, it has been our goal to place the experience of the chronic pain sufferer more squarely in the center of analytic and medical attention. We acknowledge the limitations of a book such as this for those most invested in the understanding of chronic pain—those who suffer from such pain. Some will undoubtedly feel we have substituted our own social science interests for the concerns of those in pain. Yet we remain convinced that the social theories we have drawn on have the potential to bring to light aspects of experience obscured by traditional medical or psychological theorizing. If the disaffirmation of the pain experience has roots in medical ideologies and power relations, efforts to empower those in pain should be supplemented by critical analyses of such ideologies and by efforts to refigure this mode of experience. Ultimately such a reconfiguration should yield a more humanly adequate interpretive framework, one that is more equal to the deeply vexing existential dilemmas that beset those who suffer with chronic pain and those who care for them. This book is dedicated to such an effort.

REFERENCES CITED

Bernstein, Richard J.
    1976   *The restructuring of social and political theory*. Philadelphia: University of Pennsylvania Press.
Brihaye, J., F. Loew, and H. W. Pia, eds.
    1987   *Pain: A medical and anthropological challenge*. Acta Neurochirurgica Supplementum 38. Vienna: Springer-Verlag.
Bruner, Jerome
    1990   *Acts of meaning*. Cambridge, Mass.: Harvard University Press.
Carr, David
    1986   *Time, narrative and history*. Bloomington: Indiana University Press.

Corin, Ellen
    1990   Facts and meaning in psychiatry: An anthropological approach to the lifeworld of schizophrenics. *Culture, Medicine and Psychiatry* 14:153–188.

Csordas, Tom
    1990   Embodiment as a paradigm for anthropology. *Ethos* 18:5–26.

Good, Byron J.
    1990   Medicine, rationality and experience: An anthropological perspective. 1990 Lewis Henry Morgan Lectures. University of Rochester, Rochester, New York, March 1990.

Good, Mary-Jo D., B. J. Good et al.
    1990   American oncology and the discourse on hope. *Culture, Medicine and Psychiatry* 14:59–79.

Hilbert, R.
    1984   The acultural dimensions of chronic pain: Flawed reality construction and the problem of meaning. *Social Problems* 31:365–378.

Iser, Wolfgang
    1978   *The act of reading: A theory of aesthetic response.* Baltimore: Johns Hopkins University Press.

Jackson, Michael
    1989   *Paths toward a clearing: Radical empiricism and ethnographic inquiry.* Bloomington: Indiana University Press.

Kaufman, Sharon R.
    1988   Toward a phenomenology of boundaries in medicine: Chronic illness experience in the case of stroke. *Medical Anthropology Quarterly* 2:338–354.

Kleinman, Arthur
    1986   *Social origins of distress and disease: Depression, neurasthenia, and pain in modern China.* New Haven, Conn.: Yale University Press.
    1988   *The illness narratives: Suffering, healing and the human condition.* New York: Basic Books.

Mattingly, Cheryl
    1989   Thinking with stories: Thinking and experience in a clinical practice. Ph.D. thesis, Massachusetts·Institute of Technology.

Mishler, Elliot G.
    1986   *Research interviewing: Context and narrative.* Cambridge, Mass.: Harvard University Press.

Pandolfi, Mariella
    1990   Boundaries inside the body: Women's sufferings in southern peasant Italy. *Culture, Medicine and Psychiatry* 14:255–273.

Ricoeur, Paul
    1984   *Time and narrative.* Chicago: University of Chicago Press.

Sarbin, Theodore R., ed.
    1986   *Narrative psychology: The storied nature of human conduct.* New York: Praeger.

Contributors

Paul E. Brodwin received his doctorate in Social Anthropology from Harvard University and is Assistant Professor in the Department of Anthropology, University of Wisconsin-Milwaukee. He has conducted field research on the history of French psychiatry in Senegal and on religious pluralism and healing in rural Haiti. His research on the experience of chronic pain included participant-observation with support groups for pain patients as well as longitudinal interviews with sufferers of chronic pain.

Linda Garro is Associate Professor in the Department of Community Health Sciences at the University of Manitoba. She holds a National Health Research Scholar award from Health and Welfare Canada. Her recent research and publications have centered on the representation of cultural knowledge about illness, understanding intracultural variation in cultural knowledge, and analyses of how individuals make illness treatment decisions. She has worked in Mexico and Ecuador as well as in North America with urban Americans and Canadian aboriginal peoples.

Byron J. Good is Associate Professor of Medical Anthropology in the Department of Social Medicine, Harvard Medical School, and Lecturer in the Department of Anthropology, Harvard University. He co-edited *Culture and Depression: Studies in the Anthropology and Cross-Cultural Psychiatry of Affect and Disorder* (University of California Press, 1985) with Arthur Kleinman. He is author of a forthcoming book, *Medicine, Rationality and Experience: An Anthropological Perspective* (Cambridge University Press), and Editor-in-Chief of the journal *Culture, Medicine and Psychiatry*. He has conducted research in Iran, Turkey, and the United States.

Mary-Jo DelVecchio Good is Associate Professor of Medical Sociology in the Department of Social Medicine, Harvard Medical School, and Lecturer in the Department of Sociology, Harvard University. She is Associate Editor of *Culture, Medicine and Psychiatry*. Research and publications over the past decade have focused on biomedicine as a cultural system, on the experience and meaning of illness, and on cross-national studies of medical practice and medical education. She has carried out field research in Iran and Turkey as well as the United States.

Jean E. Jackson is Professor of Anthropology and Head, Anthropology/ Archaeology Program, M.I.T. Earlier research in Mexico, Guatemala, and Colombia focused on birth spacing, anthropological linguistics, patrilineality and demography, and gender. More recent research interests include the epistemology of anthropological fieldnotes, ethnicity, indigenous rights movements, and chronic pain. She published *The Fish People: Marriage and Linguistic Identity in Northwest Amazonia* in 1983 (Cambridge University Press), and is writing a book on the pain research discussed in this volume.

Arthur Kleinman is Professor of Medical Anthropology and Psychiatry at Harvard University. His publications include *Patients and Healers in the Context of Culture* (University of California Press, 1980), *The Illness Narratives: Suffering, Healing and the Human Condition* (Basic Books, 1988), and *Rethinking Psychiatry: From Cultural Category to Personal Experience* (Free Press, 1988). He has conducted field research in Taiwan, China, and the United States.

INDEX

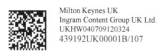
Milton Keynes UK
Ingram Content Group UK Ltd.
UKHW040709120324
439192UK00001B/107